Five Management Competency:

Building an Effective Executive Team in Behavioral Health & Social Services

An *OPEN MINDS* Publication, 2nd Edition

Edited by Monica E. Oss, M.S. & J. Jay Mackie, Ph.D.

Copyright © 2008 Behavioral Health Industry News, Inc.
Five Pillars of Management Competency: Building an Effective Executive Team in
Behavioral Health & Social Services - An *OPEN MINDS* Publication, 2nd Edition
OPEN MINDS Publication 14
ISBN 978-1-59423-141-4
Date Produced: July 28, 2008
Printed in the United States of America
OPEN MINDS, 163 York Street, Gettysburg, Pennsylvania 17325-1933
717-334-1329, fax: 717-334-0538, openminds@openminds.com, http://www.openminds.com

Five Pillars of Management Competency:
Building an Effective Executive Team in Behavioral Health & Social Services

Table of Contents

Marketing & Development Competency

Information Technology Competency

Strategic Management Competency

Contributing Authors Biographies

About *OPEN MINDS*

Five Pillars of Management Competency:
Building an Effective Executive Team in Behavioral Health & Social Services

Tables, Charts, Graphs

Is Your Team Prepared?
The Five Pillars of Management Competency in Behavioral Health & Social Services

Joseph P. Naughton-Travers, Ed.M.

Success for behavioral health and social service provider organizations is based on two key variables: 1) having the right organizational strategy, and 2) having a team with the right skills to manage the organization and implement that strategy. These characteristics constitute the infamous "doing the right things" of transformational leadership and "doing things right" of transactional leadership. The focus of this article is on the less "sexy" — but absolutely essential — transactional skills.

While there is much ado about what to do, I've seen the carnage that results when a management team is lacking some key transactional management competencies. All too typical is the situation where a major software implementation goes awry when project management and planning skills are lacking, or the failure of a new program to meet its financial targets because of a lack of supervisory and process design skills to assure that productivity levels are met. Or, the most common, the last strategic plan was never implemented because there was no performance measurement system in place to ensure progress.

So, how can we prevent operations tragedies like these? Start by knowing what the five pillars of management competency are, then conduct a gap analysis on the skills of your management team so you can figure out where improvement needs to occur.

Defining Critical Competencies

In our work at *OPEN MINDS*, we have identified five core non-clinical management competencies that behavioral health and social service organizations need in their management teams to survive and thrive in today's environment:

- Leadership and strategic planning
- Financial management
- Marketing and development capabilities
- Information technology deployment and information management
- Strategic management of operations and human capital

The first of these is really the transformational leadership competency — the leadership and planning capabilities needed to develop, communicate, and facilitate organizational vision and strategy. This includes the talent not only to develop a vision, but also to lead the organizational changes in alignment to make it succeed. Managers with this competency know when to seek out collaborations and partnerships and how to change structures and incentives, and are adept at communicating the vision to a wide set of audiences. This competency is really about being able to see the big picture, then come up with a plan to move your organization forward to be successful.

The other four competencies fall squarely in the area of transactional leadership. The financial management competencies include the ability to understand financial processes and metrics — and then to use that information to improve the organization's efficiency and effectiveness. This includes skills at analytical thinking, expert knowledge of traditional financial and business management tools (such as process improvement, unit and target costing, and return-on-investment analysis), and the ability to plan, budget, and manage complex projects and programs.

The marketing and development competencies are about the ability to communicate with and link to your organization's customer base — consumers, referral sources, payers, donors, and the local community. Managers with these competencies are experts in the "Four Ps" of marketing:

- **Product:** Designing the specifications of products and services, including what sets them apart from the competition and how they match up with the needs of customers
- **Pricing:** Establishing the price of a product or service that produces a margin and is acceptable to customers

- **Promotion:** Using tools for communicating with customers — advertising, web site, direct mail, proposal writing, and public relations for both product/service lines and the company itself
- **Place/Placement:** Addressing the way services or products reach customers, including distribution methods, geographic regions or industries, and market segments

Marketing and development competencies include the ability to develop and implement innovative services based on market demand, as well as the skills necessary to continually manage and change the organization's array of services ("service portfolio") to meet the changing needs of the marketplace.

Information technology competencies are about understanding how to use technology — and its resulting information — effectively. This includes what we call "information literacy," the ability to understand and use data to manage your organization. It also includes the ability to effectively select, plan, and deploy the use of information technologies to help the organization achieve its strategic and operational objectives.

The last category — the strategic management competencies — includes skills in both operational performance and human capital management. Operational performance management requires the ability to establish — and effectively use — performance objectives and the processes that enable staff to achieve your organizational goals. Human capital management requires the knowledge and skill to select, manage, develop, organize, and deploy your staff effectively.

Assessing Your Team

The issue of management competencies brings several key questions to mind:
- What gaps does our organization have in these critical management competencies?
- What is the potential impact of the absence of these critical skills on our success as an organization?
- What competencies do individual staff members need to develop, and how can we develop them?
- Should we "buy" the competencies (through hiring new staff members or consultants) or build them into the team we have?

The first step in answering these questions is to formally assess the core competencies of your management team. This can be done by bringing in an outside consultant or internally through a self-evaluation and group evaluation rating system. In the latter you begin by teaching your team about the basic competencies and then asking team members to rate themselves and one another on each of the competencies (typically with a simple Likert scale). You can then compile the results for individuals and the team as a whole to identify gaps and discuss a development plan.

Building Management Competency

Once you've done your competency gap analysis, you need to put together a plan to fill in the gaps. Building competencies takes time and, since competencies are enduring traits and talents, developing them takes more than just reading about them or attending classes. (However, formal education is a good start!) Competencies must be developed through training, practice, and appropriate support and feedback. Approaches may include education, coaching, or mentoring (with internal staff or outside experts) and giving staff new projects or work assignments that require them to work on the competency.

Thus, you end up with an overall staff development plan — both for your management team as a whole and for the individuals. The question then becomes "how long will it take to build the competencies we need, and can we afford to wait?" If you need the skills immediately, you will probably have to "buy" them. On a short-term basis, this would be through consultants or temporary staffing. On a longer-term basis, it would be about seeking, recruiting, and hiring new staff with the competencies that you need. Additionally — and alarmingly — there is always a risk that individual staff may not be successful in actually developing the competency you're aiming for. So, you'll need to figure out what is best for your organization — to build or buy these critical management competencies. Once you've done so, you'll know you have the organizational talent needed to execute that ambitious strategy that you've laid out. ⌘

Leadership & Planning

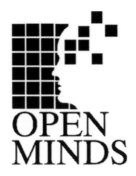

OPEN
MINDS

The Challenges & Opportunities for Human Service Management in the Next Decade

Monica E. Oss, M.S., M. Colleen Elmer, M.S.W., .M.B.A., LCSW, & John F. Talbot, Ph.D.,

Planning for the future has taken on new dimensions for most organizations in the human services field. Rapid and continuous changes in the field are the result of independent actions of political entities, health-related businesses, and non-profit organizations. The combination of recent government policy decisions, changing payer financing models, advances in service technology, and evolving consumer preference have created a unique environment for serving communities in need. Futurists looking ahead at the health and human services field predict longer life expectancy (to 110 years of age) due to medical breakthroughs that will "cure" illnesses such as cancer and heart disease. The resulting aging population will bring to the human service system higher levels of disability, bionic parts, and wired homes. These longer, technology-assisted lives will move questions of health care and social service access into sharper focus, with the likely end of employer-sponsored health care, a move to consumer-directed service systems, and the emergence of a global health and human service market.

Despite these momentous changes, today's health and human service executives have more immediate concerns. They are serving people in the here and now. This article is focused on the "here and now" and the environmental factors that will reshape the human services landscape in the decade ahead.

To understand the current human services marketplace, it is important to understand the simultaneous changes in three key environmental domains:

- Public and private payers for health and human services
- The management programs employed by payers to manage health and human service funding
- Service treatment context, including modalities and locations of service, clinical treatment models, and support service delivery systems

These three market factors are changing independently, but their evolution is synergistic — with complex intricacies between the policies of payers, the preference of consumers, and new technologies and business practices in the field.

Figure 1: Synergistic Environmental Effects on Organizational Strategy

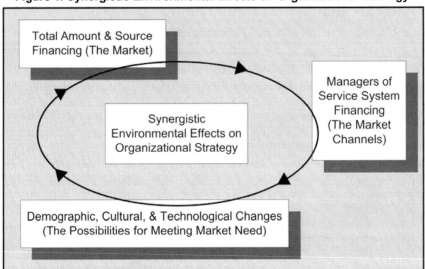

The Changing Policies & Practices of Funders of Health & Human Services

The financing of the health and human services field is changing at both the federal and state levels, and managed care's influence over costs is increasing as well. One key driver of change is federal policies designed to give states wide discretion in managing health and human services while concurrently shifting a greater portion of financial contribution to the states as well.

States have been given more flexibility and "discretion" to alter the health and human service landscape through Medicaid waivers and block grants. As a result, consumer services within the United States are increasingly varied by geography. Additionally, both the Deficit Reduction Act and Center for Medicare and Medicaid Services' Financial Integrity Rules were designed to narrow the scope of federal financing. New Medicare Advantage Special Needs Plans are also moving disabled consumers to private delivery systems. These federal policies have increased the role of the private sector in the delivery of service to disenfranchised populations and have increased the financial burden for their services on state government. As a result, states are implementing new health and human services "private sector" purchasing models to increase the "reach" of state dollars. State policymakers are also integrating funding streams to save both administrative and service dollars.

Across the health care system, managed care remains the dominant cost control mechanism in the public and private sector. Managed care enrollment in Medicaid and Medicare are on the rise while simultaneously managed care types of financing models are being adopted to intellectual and developmental disabilities through the disability care coordination concept, and managed care principles are being applied to child welfare funding through privatization initiatives and performance-based contracting. One alternative to managed care delivery models that is emerging is new consumer-directed models of care. Known as consumer-directed health plans, vouchers, health opportunity accounts, or "cash and counseling," these models will move more direct decision-making about services to consumers.

The Changing Service Delivery System

The service delivery system landscape is changing as treatment and service modalities shift and integration of services occurs at the community level. Across the country there has been a significant drop in the use of inpatient and residential services and a decreased use of nursing home-levels of service. At the same time, the use of assisted living, board-and-care homes, and foster family services is increasing. The past decade has also seen an expansion of clinic-based services and a great increase in the utilization of home and community-based services.

In addition to these shifts in modalities of care, integration of service delivery is changing. The historical structure of the health and human services field traditionally has been based on separate systems for physical health services, mental health and addiction services, and social services. A combination of payer policies and service delivery technologies are forcing these integrated service system modalities to emerge.

A few examples of the changing delivery system include:

- Behavioral health services are increasingly being delivered in primary care delivery locations and by non-psychiatric specialists
- Disability support systems and senior services delivered in long-term care settings are becoming the locus of health care delivery for residents
- More mental health services delivered within the child welfare and juvenile justice system
- Growth of the U.S. population in the adult corrections system, and the concomitant growth of behavioral health services within that setting as well as a rise in social services to support individuals leaving the system
- Educational system emerging as primary physical and behavioral health care location for many children

Across the health care system and the human services systems, addiction and mental health disorders are prominent factors in both service and system costs. For this reason, both the issue of parity and the shifts in behavioral health funding have a great effect on organizations in the field and the consumers that they serve. Overall spending in mental health and addictions treatment is on the rise, with the 2007 spending on behavioral health treatment estimated to be $148 billion. However, as spending patterns are shifting, they have serious implications for human service provider organizations. In 2003, spending for inpatient and residential services decreased to 23.5% of overall behavioral heath spending, which is down from 37.4% in 1993; conversely, outpatient spending rose slightly. The largest increase in spending was in pharmaceutical interventions, with those technologies replacing traditional "service-only" interventions.[1] These spending patterns reflect the changes at the service level and point to the new treatment models needed by service organizations in the years ahead.

---

1 Mark, T.L., R.M. Coffey, K.R. Levit, J.A. Buck, R. Vandivort-Warren Team (August 2007). Mental health treatment expenditure trends, 1986-2003. *Psychiatric Services*: vol. 58, no. 8. pgs. 1041-1048.

"Disruptive Innovations" Will Have a Significant Impact on the Delivery of Health & Human Services

The health and social service system is on the brink of significant reengineering due to recently commercialized clinical, support service, and communications technologies — technologies that will be increasingly common in the field. These technologies will have two disruptive effects on the service-system — acceptance of a broad array of less-specialized professionals to meet the needs of consumers and alluring more consumers to return home or to remain at home. For human service organizations, these technologies represent service delivery innovation that will fundamentally change their interaction with consumers as well as precipitate the re-design of service delivery.

These emerging disruptive technologies fall into five categories:
- New biomedical tools
- Technologies supporting remote service delivery
- Technologies supporting the "smart home concept"
- Technologies for cognitive retraining
- Technologies promoting consumer self-service

New Biomedical Tools

There are many forms of biomedical tools emerging that will play a large role in the delivery of health and human services. Innovative drug delivery systems — such as patches, injectables, and genetically-designed drugs — are being developed that will provide more effective and more convenient treatment. Examples of these new tools include transdermal patches for depression, long-acting injectable antipsychotic medications, and addiction substitute/blocking maintenance medications. Additionally, there has been incredible advancement in technologies used to both diagnose and treat individuals. Emerging neurotechnologies, like vagus nerve stimulation for epilepsy and deep brain stimulation for obsessive compulsive disorder and Parkinson's disease, are breakthrough non-pharmaceutical interventions for behavioral disorders. These new treatment interventions, combined with better diagnostic tools for cognitive and behavioral disorders, are changing the service delivery landscape.

Technologies Supporting Remote Service Delivery

As the Internet and wireless technology take on an increasingly prominent role in the daily lives of millions of Americans, it is logical to think that these tools of everyday living will be applied to human services. Consumers can now participate in virtual services, on-line treatment programs, remote health status monitoring, and video e-health. The same technologies are also being deployed to provide remote education, case management, and social support.

Technologies Supporting the "Smart Home Concept"

Emerging technologies have led to the creation of the "smart home" concept, aligning individuals who would previously have required nursing home placement or hospitalization to return home or remain at home. In-home activity sensors, remote health status monitoring, two-way interactive video communication, and GPS tracking are all capabilities that can be used to design a "smart home" for a consumer.

Technologies for Cognitive Retraining

Cognitive retraining is one aspect of cognitive rehabilitation — a comprehensive approach to restoring skills (such as remembering, reasoning, understanding, etc.) after brain injury or other disability. A variety of new technologies are being introduced that will increase the effectiveness and decrease the cost (and labor intensity) of cognitive retraining. Virtual reality and computer simulations are just two of many technologies being employed for conditions as diverse as anxiety disorders, attention deficit disorder, and autism.

Technologies Promoting Consumer Self-Service

A wide array of Internet-based tools are emerging that promote consumer self-service in the health and human service setting. Current tools on the market include on-line diagnostic tests, compliance monitoring, prescription ordering, appointment management, and eligibility determination.

Demographics Will Change both the Consumers and the Workforce

Changing U.S. demographics will affect both the characteristics of the consumers served and the labor supply. With regard to consumers of human services, provider organizations can expect an older consumer population with increasingly complex disabilities that accompany increased life expectancy. In addition, this population will be increasingly culturally diverse population. Similar demographic factors will affect the workforce as well. The "baby boomer" bulge is nearing retirement age, creating succession planning issues for staff at all levels. The growing demand of the aging consumer for home-based services is increasing the "competitive" wage rate for frontline staff in most markets. Foster families and home health aides, both of which are essential to the emerging delivery system, are organizing to increase their economic "clout." These labor disruptions are issues causing the proportion of organizational labor budgets spent on outsourcing, overtime, and consultants to rise.[2]

Evolving Customer Expectations

In the human service field, changing preferences are seen in both customers — payers of service and the consumers using these services.

The key driver for all payers is "value," which has led more payers to insist on better data on service delivery and effectiveness and to embrace pay-for-performance models. Sometimes termed as "rewarding excellence" or "paying for results,"[3] the ultimate and overarching goal of a pay for performance initiative is to create a direct link between financial compensation and the delivery of high quality, evidence-based, effective care.[4]

---

2 Amig, S. and M.E. Oss. (June 2001). The human capital crisis in behavioral health and social services: the implications of the new workforce demographics are widespread. *OPEN MINDS Advisor*, 3:6, 3-6.

3 Wilensky, G. (December 2005). Meeting the pay-for-performance imperative: pay for performance is one of Washington's most popular healthcare buzzwords. *Healthcare Financial Management*. Retrieved August 22, 2007 from http://findarticles.com/p/articles/mi_m3257/is_12_59/ai_n15980875#

4 Pelonero, A. L. and R.L. Johnson. (April 2007). Economic grand rounds: a pay-for-performance program for behavioral health care practitioners. *Psychiatric Services*: 58. pgs. 442-444.

The challenge of payer-defined quality measures and performance-based compensation for human services is two-fold. On the technology side, the issue is the information infrastructure needs to measure performance. But the evolution also demands moving organizational culture to one of measurement and performance enhancement.

In addition to pay-for-performance models, payers at the state and county levels are moving to more purchasing models that use some elements of risk sharing, privatization and competitive bidding.

Consumer standards are also changing in the U.S. The "consumerism" that characterizes the commercial environment has made its way to health and human services, allowing for increased consumer control of decision making opportunities about service and providing higher levels of customer service.

The Emerging Human Service Environment

The synergistic effects of these factors can be seen on the "front lines" of human service delivery. The market is evolving due to the "push" of payers to integrate services and move financial risk to other stakeholders and the "pull" of consumer preference for easy-to-use recovery-focused treatment and support services that are increasingly available and affordable with newly-created technologies. The effects of these system dynamics translate into a "perfect storm" driving a new model for change.

Taking into account all of these changes, the successful human services delivery system in five years is likely to share these characteristics:

- Integrated with other service systems (as defined by the local market)
- Able to accept risk-based and/or performance-based payment (as preferred by the local payer)
- Consumer-centric services
- Able to demonstrate a desired value proposition to consumers and local payers
- Systems in place to deliver as much home-based and community-based service as technologically feasible and preferred by the consumers and payers

These changes have several strategic implications for organizations in the field. First and foremost, there is more competition for "consumers" across the health and human service system, as well as the substitution of new technologies for traditional services.

Both create the need for executive teams to re-evaluate their service offerings. This new market environment leads to both the need for capital and an assessment of the economies of scale critical for on-going competitive success. In planning for the next decade the executive teams need to consider the changing financial underpinnings of the field, including declining fee-for-service pricing and unit cost management; inflexible "commodity" relationship with payers and their agents; and the shifting burden of uncompensated care.

The cultural and practical issues of adoption of new technologies is another critical issue; along with the investment capital and human capital needed to facilitate major organizational change. Finally, for all mission-based organizations, the board members and executives face the here-and-now challenge of balancing mission in the current financial environment.

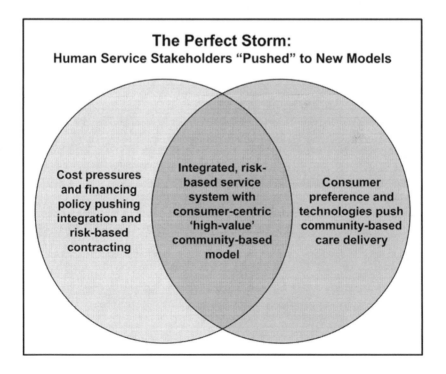

The Perfect Storm:
Human Service Stakeholders "Pushed" to New Models

Cost pressures and financing policy pushing integration and risk-based contracting

Integrated, risk-based service system with consumer-centric 'high-value' community-based model

Consumer preference and technologies push community-based care delivery

The Leadership Challenge of the Next Decade

Over the next decade, leaders in the health and human services field will need to adopt and evolve in order to deal with an evolving service delivery landscape. On a systematic level, organizations will need to deploy scenario-based planning as a tool for preparing the organization for change as needed in the local market environment. Part of this planning challenge will be to reconcile the short-term business needs of the organization in the context of the long-term vision and mission for the organization. Organizational development will also be key. The organization will need to develop executive team members' management competencies. But executives will also need enhanced transformational leadership skills — the ability to lead a plan that balances mission with the financial realities of the changing environment. With these tools and the knowledge of the upcoming trends within the health and human services field, leaders can assure their organizations continue to be a valuable community asset in the decade ahead. ▧

Changing Landscape Drives Six Key Management Initiatives: Both Business Environment & Politics Shape Behavioral Health & Social Services

Monica E. Oss, M.S. & Joseph P. Naughton-Travers, Ed.M.

> *"The essence of formulating competitive strategy is relating a company to its environment. Although the relevant environment is very broad, encompassing social as well as economic forces, the key aspect of a firm's environment is the industry or industries in which it competes."*

That's a quote by Michael E. Porter from one of his books on competitive strategy. He stresses the need for an external focus in strategic planning — tracking the major economic, political, cultural, and technological changes that will have the greatest impact on our organizations, and determining how to achieve our mission and objectives amidst them.

In the behavioral health and social service field, there are two major environmental forces driving change — (1) a changing framework — political, cultural, and technological — in which organizations operate, and (2) significant changes occurring in the available health and human services resources in the United States — and the rules for using those resources are shifting.

With regard to the changing framework within which our organizations operate, we are encountering changing demands from our customers, improved psychotropic medications and new technologies, and shifting population demographics. The changes in resources and resource rules — from strapped Medicaid budgets and state funds to privatization and managed care — are the subject of daily newspaper articles.

This article is designed to synthesize the latest available information about the behavioral health and social service landscape, and to discuss the management initiatives that have developed in response.

The Changing Political, Cultural & Technological Framework in the United States

A complex set of factors has fundamentally changed the operating environment for all organizations (not just those in our field). The most striking is the "new consumerism" in the U.S. — consumers' interest in customization, convenience, and speed. Organizations in our field serve an array of customers — service funders (both public and employer-based), consumers and their families, and care management organizations. Each set of customers has its own unique demands, service expectations, and definitions of value. On the payer front, we continue to see a trend towards performance measurement by both public and private purchasers as a way to ensure value. In some jurisdictions, payment for services is linked to performance through bonus and penalty systems in provider and managed care organization contracting.

On the consumer side, consumers and their families now play a more active role than ever in behavioral health and social service planning. They define positive outcomes in terms of social and functional measures (such as the abilities to maintain jobs, relationships, and a home) rather than the clinical outcomes that professionals previously used to define value and quality. The "new consumerism" in our field has several key components:

- Demand for choice in treatment options and care providers
- Desire for more control and independent functioning through self-care and self- management? Requirement to play an active role in treatment planning and decision-making ("consumer-directed care")
- Expectation for better "customer service" when receiving services
- Demand for access to health care information (now formalized under HIPAA privacy standards)

In addition to changing customer expectations, behavioral health and social service organizations now have to consider the competitive advantages of new biomedical, information, and telecommunication technologies. The emergence of state-of-the industry psychotropic medications has been both a blessing and a challenge. In the year 2000 alone, the Federal Drug Administration (FDA) approved over 70 new psychotropic medications. We've seen enormous benefit from these new drugs — improved functioning as well as reduced side effects and service costs. However, the higher per consumer costs of these new medications are creating tension in how health care services are financed and what services are purchased. This tension is particularly dramatic in markets where medications are covered by one payer or funding stream and behavioral health services by another.

We continue to see the rapid evolution and adoption of information system and telecommunication technologies. While behavioral health and social service organizations have generally been slower to implement these new technologies (and still spend less per employee on them than nearly all other industries), the array of choices is growing:

- Practice management software to increase administrative efficiencies and manage service operations
- Care management software with core functionality for service authorization, claims processing, and provider network management
- Electronic medical record capabilities
- Outcomes measurement software
- Wireless technologies for communication, data entry, and information access
- Telehealth technologies, including internet and video-based service delivery
- On-line interactive consumer services for self-help and community support

The last component of the changing environmental framework in which we do business is population demographics. The 2000 census revealed a continued shift in the demographics of the U.S. population — affecting both the consumers we serve and the staff we employ. Overall, the population is aging and becoming increasingly diverse in terms of race and ethnicity. The workforce includes more women, and employees increasingly seek better balances between their work and family lives. Additionally, with the availability of the new psychotropic medications, we are seeing more behavioral health consumers who were previously unemployed working in our organizations.

Reduced Resources & New "Resource Rules"

In addition to changes in the environment framework, there are significant changes in the available financial resources for behavioral health and social services and the rules for using those resources. We are in the midst of national economic downturn with state budget deficits across the nation. To further complicate the matter, health care expenditures continue to grow in both the public and private sector, forcing payers to figure out how to do more with less.

For years, states have tried to combat the problem of rising health care budgets by working hard to increase the share of federal reimbursement for health care expenditures. They do this by "maximizing Medicaid" — that is, seeking to qualify the services under the Medicaid program because it includes a federal match to state spending. The strategy worked. Federal funds are now used to pay for more than 50% of public mental health services in the United States, and by the year 2017, it is estimated that Medicaid will pay nearly 70% of states' budgets for mental health services.

This shift towards Medicaid financing of behavioral health services is changing how services are purchased as well as what consumers are served. The federal procurement guidelines that Medicaid uses are resulting in more competitive bidding for selection of both public and private care management and service provider organizations. The increased use of Medicaid waivers affects consumer choice, use of financial risk transfer mechanisms, and the overall service benefit packages covered in the state healthcare plans. Overall, the public mental health system is changing from a "safety net" for citizens to a system focused on using definitions of Medicaid eligibility and medical necessity to determine who receives services. This has obvious implications for county-based and private service provider organizations. But there are even bigger implications for employers — no more "free service" for employed individuals with poor health insurance benefits.

In addition to the shift to increased Medicaid funding of services, many states are seeking to "blend" their various funding streams so that resources are pooled and consumer-focused. The belief is that this will result in better care coordination, reduced cost-shifting between public agencies, and reduced overall service and administrative costs. This occurs most commonly in two instances: (1) blending mental health and substance abuse service funds for adults; and (2) blending funds for services for children and youth (including Medicaid, child welfare, juvenile justice, and/or special education funds). Blended funding has many benefits, but behavioral health and social service provider organizations are encountering increased complexity in billing as they cope with multiple payer requirements for documentation of services. Clinical staff — particularly at child welfare agencies — wrestle with increased medical record documentation requirements in order to comply with the various payer standards.

At the same time that blended funding models are evolving, privatization, competitive bidding, and managed care models for behavioral health services have become commonplace. The number of states with managed behavioral health programs tripled in the period 1996 to 1999. Based on 1999 data, fully fifty-six percent of Medicaid and Medicare enrollees were covered under a managed care plan. At this point in time, 30 states have Title IV-E waivers in place to allow them to use funds for placement services for children more flexibly, and there are 47 different managed care initiatives in child welfare underway.

Lastly, we note a growing demand for publicly financed behavioral health services. This has resulted both from increasing unemployment and the lack of parity in health insurance. More U.S. citizens are uninsured — either because they are unemployed altogether or because they are contract employees or temporary workers, and many individuals with serious mental illness are "under-insured." Both groups wind up being served by our public behavioral health system.

Strategic Implications for Executives & Managers

The current environmental trends pose both challenges and opportunities for behavioral health and social service organizations. While declining resources and the economic situation pose a gloomy picture, entrepreneurial organizations can find ways to leverage new technologies and restructure their organizations to successfully compete for both contracts and consumers. Executives in the field are employing six strategies to cope with the changing landscape:
- Maximizing the use of strategic and operational performance metrics
- Leveraging information and telecommunication technologies
- Enhancing costing and financial management operations
- Enhanced human resource management
- Retooling clinical service delivery
- Planning for consolidation, collaborations, centralization, and mergers

1. Maximizing the Use of Strategic & Operational Performance Metrics

Behavioral health and social services organizations are implementing broad approaches to performance measurement and reporting in order to meet customer demands and manage quality and cost in uncertain economic times. These performance measurement systems incorporate metrics based on customer definitions of value and quality as well as critical operational measures. Successful organizations have the infrastructure and trained staff to manage these metrics and to use the information on service line development and strategies that focus on consumer-defined quality attributes.

2. Leveraging Information & Telecommunication Technologies

Most organizations have needed to considerably increase their investments in technologies and the infrastructure and staff needed to support them in order to meet the information demands of both internal and external constituencies and to streamline and automate operations. Electronic medical records, wireless devices, telehealth services, and Internet-based education and support services will all play a critical role in controlling cost. Formal return-on-investment (ROI) analyses are being used to determine the costs and savings associated with these technologies to aid in decision-making.

3. Enhancing Costing & Financial Management Operations

Payers — federal, state, and private — continue to demand greater cost controls as well as demonstration of value in services being purchased. As a result, behavioral health and social service organizations need to "do more with less" in order to survive. This means these organizations need new financial management competencies — unit-cost reporting and management, enhanced third-party billing skills, and target cost-based product development and pricing systems. For many organizations, achieving these competencies has required new (or different) staff and information systems.

4. Enhanced Human Resource Management

Just as with financial management, behavioral health and social service organizations must increase their focus on human resource management in order to ensure they can recruit and retain high-quality staff. New staff development programs are focusing on critical areas of competency — leadership, financial management, strategic management, marketing development, and the use of technology. The ability to recruit a multi-lingual, culturally sensitive workforce is critical to success with an increasingly diverse population, and organizations whose workforce does not reflect the diversity of the population find it more difficult to compete. Human resource departments will need to focus extensively on the issues of diversity, work life, and compensation arrangements.

5. Retooling Clinical Service Delivery

Clinical service delivery systems are being transformed from admission to discharge. Clinical staff and the treatment planning systems they use need to embrace both evidence-based treatment practices and consumer demand for "customer service" with an active role in treatment. There is a strong push to demonstrate the cost offsets of psychotropics, to demonstrate customer-defined outcomes, and to develop evidence-based formularies. Provider organizations have found they need additional psychiatric and nursing staff to support medication evaluation and management operations. Telehealth and Internet-based professional and consumer support services are also being embraced as adjuncts to face-to-face service delivery.

6. Planning for Consolidation, Collaboration, Centralization & Mergers

Size and economies of scale remain critical strategic issues for behavioral health and social service organizations. Smaller organizations are not able to afford the technological and human resource investments needed for success, nor are they able to gain required efficiencies to control cost without strategic alliances. Consolidation, centralization, and mergers will be key to survival and success in the industry. ▣

Leadership & Planning Competency

Making the Most of a SWOT Analysis: Use This Standard Tool to Identify "Best Fit" Opportunities

Monica E. Oss, M.S.

The SWOT analysis methodology has been used by a broad range of organizations over the years. Essentially, a SWOT analysis is a basic management tool that identifies the Strengths, Weaknesses, Opportunities, and Threats of an organization and helps in assessing environmental factors as internal strengths and weaknesses and external opportunities and threats. The reason for the staying power of the SWOT analysis is that this technique:

- Is easy to use
- Combines both quantitative and qualitative analysis
- Encourages interdepartmental collaboration
- Helps to focus large amounts of information into manageable amounts for analysis

Frankly, I have been fairly negative about using SWOT analysis until recently. The first problem with SWOT is that the process really only works when you can be brutally honest about your organization — which is sometimes difficult for even the most progressive organizations. The second is that SWOT analysis falls short of providing "next steps" in the process — strategies for addressing the strengths, weaknesses, opportunities, and threats that you have identified.

The lack of objectivity can be addressed by using a facilitator from outside the organization or involving external experts in the process. The strategic implications can be overcome by using a structured process in creating and analyzing the SWOT data. While models vary, the process I recommend has four steps:

1. Prepare a preliminary executive team assessment of SWOT factors.
2. Build on the executive team assessment with members of the board and/or outside subject matter expert(s).
3. Use a nominal voting process to prioritize the factors.

4. Based on the high priority factors, develop strategies to address both internal and external circumstances.

This process has worked successfully for a number of behavioral health and social services organizations.

Prepare a Preliminary Executive Team Assessment

The SWOT analysis begins with a systematic inventory of your organization's strengths, weaknesses, opportunities, and threats. Strengths and weaknesses are the internal core competencies and resources that are under your organization's control. Opportunities and threats are external factors over which you have no immediate control. Prior to the executive team SWOT meeting, have each participant spend some time considering all of these factors and preparing a preliminary assessment of the organizational SWOT. These lists, generated by your executive team, will form the basis of the group discussion.

SWOT Matrix	
Strengths	**Weaknesses**
List 4-5 internal strengths 1. 2. 3. 4. 5.	List 4-5 internal weaknesses 1. 2. 3. 4. 5.
Opportunities	**Threats**
List 4-5 external opportunities 1. 2. 3. 4. 5.	List 4-5 external threats 1. 2. 3. 4. 5.

Strengths and Weaknesses

An organization's internal strengths and weaknesses are rooted in many tangible and intangible aspects. They are internal elements affecting the organization and are evaluated based on honest and realistic assessment of a number of factors.

The designation of strength or weakness will be based on the answers to questions such as:

- What are the organization's financial reserves, physical assets, and/or on-going contracts?
- Are we on the "plus side" in terms of revenue and margin?
- Are administrative costs in line with revenues?
- What are our core competencies? Significant areas of experience and/or expertise?
- What role do location and geography play in our organization?
- What is the status of our accreditations and certifications?
- What is the state of our infrastructure, such as information technology, communications, and billing systems?
- How strong is our leadership? Do we have a succession plan in place?
- Does the organization have a clear internal vision and mission?
- What are our key staffing capabilities and human capital/resources?
- What is our staff turnover rate?
- What is our corporate culture? How healthy are our internal working relationships?
- How prepared are we to deal with change in the environment? How innovative are we?
- What do we do better than anyone else? And does it matter to our customers?
- How effective is our documentation? How well do we keep clinical records?
- Are our outcomes quantifiable and objectively measurable? Do we have evidence-based practices in place?
- What level of consumer satisfaction do we achieve? What about customer satisfaction?

Opportunities and Threats

The analysis of external factors requires time for data-gathering and reflection — but this information is absolutely crucial for a successful analysis. Be sure to consider carefully all the forces that are "in play" and affecting the marketplace and your organization's place within it. These external factors, which are outside your organization's control, can be either opportunities or threats, based on the answers to questions such as:

- Are the needs of our customers changing?
- Are our competitors increasing their market share?
- What market trends are affecting the market place?
- How are our business partners affected by changes in the environment
- Does our association with them pose opportunities or threats?
- What political or social issues affect our organization?
- What economic factors (such as labor costs or recession, etc.) are occurring that affect us?
- What technological developments will impact our business?
- What legislative or regulatory changes or issues are on the horizon?

In each case, the external factors present either opportunities or threats to your organization, and it is not always immediately apparent which is which.

Build on the Executive Team Assessment With Members of the Board and/or Outside Subject Matter Expert(s)

The next step in the process, once the executive team has made independent lists of strengths, weaknesses, opportunities, and threats, is to conduct a group "brainstorming" session with the executive team, members of the board, and including external experts. The goal of the brainstorming session is to add as many items as possible to the preliminary executive team assessment. This can be done in a morning session, using white boards or flip charts to record suggestions as they are made. It is important to allow adequate time for discussion. This is where the services of an outside facilitator can be particularly helpful in moving a "myopic" discussion to a productive one.

Use a Nominal Voting Process to Prioritize the Factors

As a next step, you need to sort our your "laundry list" of items and prioritize those that are most mission critical. One technique I've used as a facilitator is to create a "SWOT Analysis Ballot." Using a nominal voting process, each member of the group can cast a fixed number of votes in each category on one or more of the identified factors. After a tally, you have your executive team's assessment of the organization's most important strengths, weaknesses, threats, and opportunities.

Based on the High Priority Factors, Develop Strategies to Address Both Internal and External Circumstances

The last and most important step is to prioritize the strategies for your organization, based on the highest priority factors. There are essentially four strategy types:

SWOT Strategic Analysis		
	Strengths	**Weaknesses**
Opportunities	**S-O Strategy Examples** Expand globally Increase sales staff Increase advertising Develop new products Diversify	**W-O Strategy Examples** Joint Venture Acquire competitor Expand nationally Backward integration Forward integration
Threats	**S-T Strategy Examples** Diversify Acquire competitor Liquidate Expand locally Re-engineer	**W-T Strategy Examples** Divest Increase promotion Retrench Restructure Downsize

- S-O strategies pursue opportunities that match and build on your organization's strengths. Examples include expanding to a new state, increasing sales staff, or developing new service lines. These are the best strategies to employ, but many organizations are not in a position to do so. This should lead to a discussion of resources required for growth.
- W-O strategies are those that are used to overcome weaknesses to pursue specific opportunities. For example, forming a joint venture to create a continuum of care for a particular customer.
- S-T strategies identify ways that an organization can use its strengths to reduce its vulnerability to external threats; for instance, expanding to a new location to take advantage of customer relationships in that geographic area and protect the customer contract from competition.

- W-T strategies establish a defensive plan to prevent an organization's weaknesses from making it susceptible to external threats, such as downsizing or restructuring the organization to meet customer needs while keeping costs at a minimum.

The resulting list of strategies to be explored becomes the backbone of the planning discussion. You may be surprised at what you discover through this process — things that seem threatening at first often turn out to be golden opportunities for organizations that recognize and act upon them. ▦

Financial Management

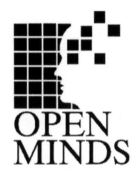

OPEN
MINDS

The New Role of the CFO in Behavioral Health & Social Services: Evolving Financial Management Role Driven by Changes in External Environment

Monica E. Oss, M.S.

Changes in the external environment of the behavioral health and social service field have changed the role of the chief financial officer (CFO). Due to a series of recent public policy decisions, the field has moved from a "cost plus" environment with limited competition, to one with increasing competition for revenues and the shifting of entitlements through capitation and global budgets. This shift in market model, used to fund behavioral health and social services, has created the need for proactive financial management integrated in all aspects of organizational strategy.

Some of the recent developments that are changing financial management needs of organizations are payer's use of market-rate and risk-based financing techniques with competitive procurement practices; new payer demands for performance measurement and contracting; the emergence of new technologies; and increasing regulatory and compliance issues. As a result, executive teams now need a strategic plan that is developed within the context of the financial metrics of market rates, limited funding, and zero-based budgets. In addition, organizations also need organization-wide approaches to performance measurement; flexible costing/billing systems that can assimilate performance-derived payment models; technology development that is integrated with planning for new services; and real-time unit cost analysis and opportunity cost analysis. Most of these new requirements fall squarely in the office of the financial officer — and many CFOs are unprepared, by either lack of education or experience, to lead these initiatives.

There are many variations to the specific organizational requirements of the CFO. However, most organizations in the field share the need to expand the role of the financial officer in five key areas:

- Integration of financial functions through the organization's operations
- Use of financial metrics (both internal and external) in developing organizational strategy
- Development and implementation of strategic performance measurement
- Rate setting and unit/case cost analysis
- Evaluation and reengineering of organizational processes

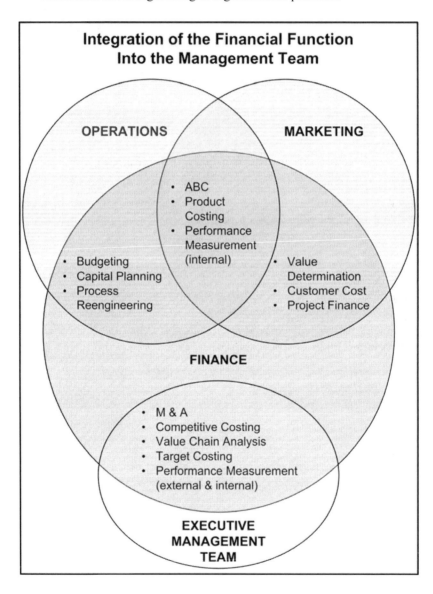

Integration of the Financial Function Into the Management Team

OPERATIONS

MARKETING

- ABC
- Product Costing
- Performance Measurement (internal)

- Budgeting
- Capital Planning
- Process Reengineering

- Value Determination
- Customer Cost
- Project Finance

FINANCE

- M & A
- Competitive Costing
- Value Chain Analysis
- Target Costing
- Performance Measurement (external & internal)

EXECUTIVE MANAGEMENT TEAM

Integration of Financial Functions Through the Organization's Operations

In a highly regulated, cost-plus environment, financial functions are largely retrospective — recording of costs, auditing, and reporting. In a less regulated and more competitive environment, financial management functions are more proactive and, by necessity, more integrated with other organizational functions. Integration of finance with marketing and operations is key in areas such as product costing, process reengineering, new product development, budgeting, and pricing. In support of the executive leadership, the CFO has new responsibilities — analysis of competitive pricing and service line positioning, target costing, organizational performance measurement, and merger/acquisition analysis.

Use of Financial Metrics in Developing Organizational Strategy

The evolving environment for financing of behavioral health and social services has led organizations to a new model of strategic planning. The model that is most effective in the new environment is goal-oriented; focused on organizational market position; integrated with planning for technology; and based on financial metrics from within and outside the organization. In the new strategic planning model, the CFO has three key roles - providing internal and external data about organizational costs and competitive rates; analyzing the position of the organization within the field with regard to market value and economies of scale; and leading the organization's budgeting process.

The analysis of organizational market position is particularly new to CFOs in the behavioral health and social service team. The questions that typically arise in the planning process are:

- How is the financing and delivery system structure of our field changing?
- In the context of these changes, how does our organization compare to its competitors?
- To achieve our objectives, do we need to focus on positioning on cost or some other factor?
- Do we need to diversify into other markets?

- As the field evolves, does our organization need to consider adopting forward/backward integration, strategic alliances, or mergers in order to survive?

Value chain analysis is one of many tools used by CFOs to answer these questions and contribute to organizational understanding of the financial metrics of the field.

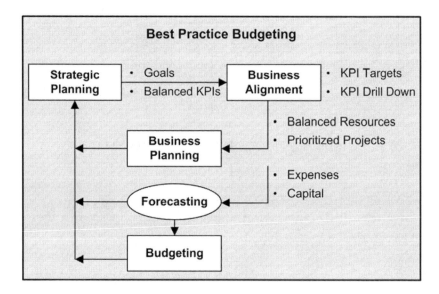

Development & Implementation of Strategic Performance Measurement

Another critical CFO role is to lead the organization's initiative to develop, monitor, and analyze the organization's measures of strategic performance. These key performance indicators (KPIs) are important measures of both the organization's success in implementing its strategic plan and the success of the organization's strategy. Much has been written about the development of KPI and models for selecting both leading and lagging financial and non-financial indicators of performance.

The challenge, beyond selecting the measures, is two-fold:
- Developing the ability to routinely report the measures using data from existing information systems (or expanding current information systems to collect the data).

- Analyzing the KPI each month and developing organizational strategies to improve problem performance.

Rate Setting & Unit/Case Cost Analysis

Rate setting and cost analysis may seem like traditional responsibilities for an organization's CFO, but these functions have evolved in a more competitive environment. In many jurisdictions, payment for behavioral health and social services is moving from cost-based payment rates to fee schedules and/or competitive procurement processes, even for organizations whose positioning is not based on cost-competitiveness; service rates and service costs matter.

Some of the questions to be answered by the CFO in assessing rates and costs include:

- What is our competitor's "market rates" for each type of service that our organization provides?
- What is our organization's actual cost of delivering each type of service?
- Given the current competitive market rates and our actual service delivery cost, does our organization need to set a different target cost? And, if so, do we need to reengineer the processes that we use to deliver these services?

Evaluation & Reengineering of Organizational Processes

Last but not least, the CFO also needs to lead organizational initiatives to evaluate organizational processes and, where necessary, reengineer those processes. Reengineering of processes can occur to address target cost issues, to adopt new technologies (both information systems and biomedical), or to improve the flow of services for consumers. There are a wide variety of methodologies and tools for process reengineering available to CFOs. Regardless of the tools selected, questions typically addressed in the reengineering process include:

- Why is this process conducted by our organization?
- What specific activities are part of this process?
- Are any of these activities specifically required by a customer?

- Could any activities be eliminated without having an impact on customers' perception of the value of the service?
- Does technology exist to eliminate any of these activities?
- Could any activities be eliminated if some prior activities were done differently?
- Are any of these activities ones for which customers are willing to pay an additional fee?

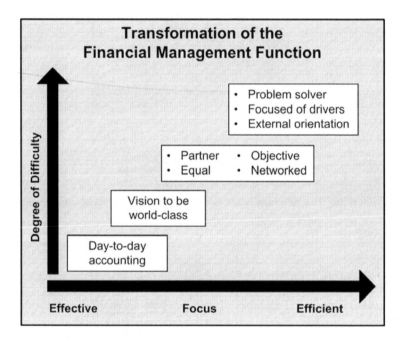

The Transition to a New Model for Financial Management

In most behavioral health and social service organizations, the role of the CFO currently has two functions — managing internal financial controls and the routine financial transactions and processes of the organization. These organizations need to develop a strategy to move the role of the CFO from day-to-day accounting functions to one of an externally oriented problem solver. The long-term vision for the organization within this changing environment is a key component in visualizing this new financial management role. ▨

Financial Management Competency

Approaching the Financial Turnaround Process: Planning for the Financial Revitalization of a Behavioral Health Organization

Niels T. Eskelsen, M.B.A., C.P.A.

At some time every organization will face the challenges of a financial turnaround. Some are preventable; some are not. And depending on your organization's funding mix, the affects of a downturn in business cycle will vary greatly. In the behavioral health and social service field, a financial turnaround has more to do with service delivery than financial reporting. Because individual financial decisions made at every level affect the whole organization, the resolution of financially revitalizing a behavioral health program requires more than a simple fix or a restatement of financial transactions.

Financial turnarounds are never comfortable or easy. The longer it takes an organization to recognize a financial crisis, the more difficult the turnaround challenge. When appropriate actions are delayed or inappropriate actions are implemented, more severe or emergent actions are necessary and the question becomes, "Why delay in taking action to prevent a financial problem?" The simple answer is that perceived barriers to a successful turnaround often appear too great for the organization's leadership. We sometimes set up rules or relationships that can not be changed. For example, barriers can be cultural, i.e. internal practices or beliefs, a lack of leadership or vision, a lack of technical or professional expertise, or a lack of willingness to take responsibility for the present situation. The basics of a successful financial turnaround are to make an honest assessment of the situation, develop a reasonable plan addressing the issues driving the financial problems, implement the plan throughout the whole organization, and diligently follow-up.

An essential component of managerial responsibility is to operate a financially viable organization. In behavioral health, financial issues are often relegated to the finance department or the chief financial officer, when in fact, operating a financially viable organization is a total management responsibility. Clinical managers have more impact over the financial viability than financial managers after all the clinical work has been done. It's this synergy between financial management and clinical management that is needed for a turnaround.

In assessing and developing a turnaround plan the easiest step is identifying the critical changes that must be achieved to correct the situation. Nearly 90% of the time critical issues can be identified by internal staff. The remaining issues may require outside consultation. Regardless, the success of a turnaround falls on the shoulders of the management team.

A financial turnaround touches every aspect of an organization. First, we must consider the preventative or early warning tools that can assist in identifying financial concerns. And then we need to identify the key issues that need to be addressed when a financial turnaround is recognized.

Early Warning Signs

Financial indicators are essential components of an early warning system. An array of indicators can be used, some as early warning indicators and some as lagging or confirming indictors. First, look at your review process. Do you review your financial indicators on a monthly basis? If not, why? If you have identified financial indicators, their implementation and use are an absolute must for any financial turnaround. The important indicators will vary depending on the nature of the program and the nature of the organization's core services. Overall organizational profitability indicators include the following:

- Agency profit actual versus budget
- Revenue and expense actual versus budget
- Program level revenue and expense actual versus budget

These indicators are suggested for three reasons. First, they are simple, easy to understand, and easy to convert into trend data. Looking at trends is actually more important than looking at single numbers. Trends tell a story over a period of time and indicate an overall direction of performance. Second, in a financial turnaround, managers must focus on financial performance, which includes increasing revenue, while maintaining and/or reducing costs. Third, each set includes an indicator that is performance related, such as, clinician productivity or bed days billed. In a financial turnaround, what matters most is the ability to generate revenues in relation to cost not focus on just being busy.

The Cash Flow Worksheet

One tool that can provide important data for preventing and/or managing a financial turnaround is the Cash Flow Worksheet. This pragmatic tool is both simple to develop and easy to maintain.

Cash flow statements are required for financial reporting. However, this type of cash flow worksheet is not very useful for your needs. The most useful tool is one developed in an Excel worksheet that shows actual cash income and cash outgoes on a weekly basis. The worksheet should be a reasonable short-term predictor of your cash balance. In the example worksheet, there is not enough cash in Week 3 to cover payroll. This allows financial managers to work with clinical managers in planning cash disbursements over time so there is a balance between cash income and cash outgo.

The Cash Flow Worksheet					
	Actual Week 1	Week 2	Week 3	Week 4	Week 5
Beginning Cash	$10,000				
Cash Income:					
Revenue Source A	$143,000	—	—	$75,000	—
Revenue Source B	—	$50,000	—	—	$55,000
Revenue Source C	—	—	$15,000	—	$50,000
Total Revenue	$143,000	$50,000	$15,000	$75,000	$105,000
Cash Disbursements:					
Payroll	$100,000	—	$100,000	—	$100,000
Taxes	$25,000	—	$25,000	—	$25,000
Rent	$5,000	—	—	—	$5,000
Utilities	$4,000	—	—	—	$4,000
Interest	—	$2,500	—	—	—
Total	$134,000	$2,500	$125,000	—	$134,000
Net Cash:	$9,000	$47,500	($110,000)	$75,000	($29,000)
Ending Cash:	$19,000	$66,500	($43,500)	$31,500	$2,500

You might say, "This is too simple!" However, in the dozen or so financial turnarounds I have managed, my first step is always gaining control over the cash by building this simple spreadsheet. From this spreadsheet, financial executives can manage the timing of cash flows while operational managers can focus on increasing cash income and managing cash outgo within their program's financial constraints. The ability to sustain long-term service delivery is dependent on how successful an organization is in not only maintaining sustaining cash flow but in building appropriate cash reserves.

Issues When Conducting a Financial Turnaround

The success of a financial turnaround is not based solely on counting money and crunching numbers. Rather, several key issues involving strategy, leadership, and organizational culture need to be considered:

- Categorize strategies by long- and short-term goals
- Find the balance between mission and margin
- Listen to customer feedback, and make immediate corrective actions to resolve all issues impacting customer relationships
- Use expense reduction as well as other strategies when implementing a turnaround
- Focus on the data that matters
- Institute a culture of accountability

Categorize Strategies by Long- and Short-Term Goals

Long-term strategies should be part of the on-going strategic planning process. Their implementation should be monitored to assure management that the organization is achieving its objectives. However, long-term strategies can become a huge distraction and be counter productive when short-term actions are required. A good long-term revenue diversification strategy is to develop a new service outside the organization's core function. However, if there is a short-term cash flow issue, this decision will divert cash away from its core business, as well as tax management time and resources. Since long-term strategies take longer to develop, implement, and mature, they should be funded either with excess funds or with revenues (i.e., donations, grants, or other non-service revenues) that have been generated for that purpose.

Short-term strategies are those that have an immediate financial (cash) impact. Ranging from one to six months, short-term strategies are those that are implemented to make immediate reductions in cost, to expand existing services to current customers, or to offer core services to new customers. Choosing the right strategy at the right time is critical.

Find the Balance Between Mission and Margin

In a financial turnaround, their must be a margin for there to be a mission. However, the values that drive some high margins may not be compatible to fulfilling your organization's mission. Take great care in delivering an acceptable quality of services within the cost constraints while satisfying your customers.

Listen to Customer Feedback, and Make Immediate Corrective Actions to Resolve All Issues Impacting Customer Relationships

Customer satisfaction may be an early indicator about how the organization is doing.

Use Expense Reduction as Well as Other Strategies When Implementing a Turnaround

While cost cutting should be part of the process, take care not to cut the cost of needed expertise or leadership that will diminish your organization's ability to sustain existing revenue, satisfy your customers, or grow promising programs.

Focus on the Data That Matters

Determine up front what your success will look like and what data will tell you when you have achieved success. You don't have to measure everything; you only need to measure the few performance indicators that tell if your plan is working.

Institute a Culture of Accountability

Senior managers must hold themselves and their staff responsible for their individual and collective performance. If the agency leadership is unwilling to make the expense reductions, alter service delivery preferences, or hold staff accountable for performance, then a financial turnaround will not happen.

At some point every organizational will face a financial turnaround. The good news is that the right tools can assist managers in managing cash and identifying trends before serious financial problems occur. However, tools are only as good as those that use them. At the close of day, it's the management team that decides an organization's ultimate future. ⧈

New Environmental Challenges Demand Better Financial Information Systems: Steps in Ensuring the Success of New Financial Systems

Joseph P. Naughton-Travers, Ed.M.

Finance departments in behavioral health and social service organizations are undergoing dramatic changes. In markets with declining revenues and margins, increasing demand for performance measurement, and greater fiscal accountability, organizations are finding that their finance departments need new competencies for success, along with more robust information systems to support business decision-making.

A new priority for the chief financial officer (CFO) and the finance department is to empower people with better and more readily available management information. For managers and line staff, real-time access to easy-to-interpret information, including combined financial and operational data, supports timely management intervention and course correction when problems arise. Senior management also requires summary financial and performance data and analysis for strategic planning, performance measurement, and adoption of new management methods. The CFO's first task, in concert with the entire organization, is to distill from the sea of data, the information needed to support good decision making.

The responsibilities of finance staff have moved well beyond the historical tasks of issuing financial statements, developing budgets, and managing accounts receivable, payroll, and payables. These new responsibilities include:

- Advanced cost accounting, including unit cost analysis and management
- Business unit, service line, and sub-corporation (if applicable) budgeting and financial reporting in addition to organization-wide consolidated financial reporting
- Product development budgeting and target costing
- Strategic and operational performance measurement and reporting
- Payer performance and cost reporting

All of these responsibilities require robust financial and management accounting information system capabilities. So, how state of the art is our field with regard to financial management systems?

In terms of practice management, managed care organization (MCO), and electronic medical software applications, we've come a long way. Most behavioral health and social service organizations have scrutinized their business needs in these areas and made comprehensive investments in these technologies and the management systems necessary to support them. Yet, in almost all instances, accounting and general ledger applications are maintained as separate software applications and organizational business needs with regards to finance have taken a back seat. In fact, many organizations are still using antiquated or legacy G/L packages with minimal financial and management accounting capabilities.

As far as vendor product offerings go, some practice management system vendors do offer turnkey or enterprise systems, but it is rare to find a vendor who can provide and maintain "best of breed" functionality in the accounting and financial management modules that supplement their core product's functionality. Other vendors tackle the integration problem by developing strategic partnerships with established financial management information system companies, offering system interfaces between the applications as a means of combining clinical, service, and financial data for analysis and reporting.

What's Different About Selecting a Financial Management Information System

Financial management information systems usually offer organizations functionality in the following key categories:
- Accounts receivable (usually in summary format, since detailed accounts receivable are resident in practice management systems)
- Accounts payable
- Asset accounting
- General ledger
- Budgeting
- Cash management and forecasting
- Cost accounting

- Payroll and human resource management
- Financial reporting (by product line and in consolidated format)

While there has been considerable attention in the industry to best practices for selecting practice management and MCO software applications, it's important to note that there are considerable differences when selecting a financial management information system. These differences include:

- Smaller number of end users, with more computer experience and clearly defined business needs
- More stable and established vendors
- Reseller sales and support model
- Established import/export capabilities

Smaller Number of End Users, With More Computer Experience and Clearly Defined Business Needs

While nearly all staff members will receive reports generated from financial management systems, there are usually considerably fewer end-users of these applications in comparison to practice management and MCO systems. Financial management systems are used almost exclusively by finance department staff, and fortunately, these are usually the staff with the greatest amount of experience and ease in using computers. Additionally, the functional business needs and "best practices" for setting up software are more clearly defined in the area of finance when compared to the other operational areas in behavioral health and social service organizations.

What does all this mean? Essentially, that selecting and implementing a financial management information system is likely to be easier than with a practice management or MCO system. It involves fewer staff, who have focused functional needs and considerable comfort and experience with software applications.

More Stable and Established Vendors

While there are several practice management system vendors who have been in business long-term, there have also been numerous companies and applications that have come and gone in recent years. With financial management information systems, the market is more mature and established, and systems have been sold to tens of thousands of users in all industries. This results in less concern about the financial viability of the software vendor, yet perhaps greater concern about its knowledge of our industry and its ability to provide customer support.

Reseller Sales and Support Model

Nearly all of the major financial management information system vendors sell their software, implementation, and support services through resellers or "certified" vendors. Essentially, this means that the system selection process should not only include appropriate due diligence (financially and operationally) of the software company, but also of the reseller or certified vendor. It is this party that really becomes your information system partner and who needs to undergo the greatest degree of scrutiny.

Established Import/Export Capabilities

Lastly, all the financial management information systems have established capabilities for importing and exporting data. The challenge in devising an integrated information reporting plan is to ensure that your practice management systems or MCO systems can "talk" to the financial management systems and to structure the table configuration files in both systems so that they are compatible.

Selecting a New System

The first step in selecting and implementing a new financial management information system is the same best practice as in any system selection — determining the essential business functionality your organization needs. Start with a review of the major categories of financial system functionality listed earlier in this article. Are there new or better capabilities that your organization needs to accomplish key operational and strategic objectives? What are the limitations and problems with your current accounting and G/L software application? What are the essential reports that staff need to manage their respective areas of responsibility?

With financial management information systems, the second step in the selection process is to make sure that you don't already have a system that does what you need! If your organization currently uses one of the more well-known applications, it is important to find out whether software upgrades or additional modules will meet your enhanced functional specifications. Or does the general ledger chart of accounts or other key table files simply need to be reconfigured in order to meet new reporting and analysis requirements? Have you spoken with a certified support vendor (or found another one if necessary) to ensure you are maximizing your use of the application?

If you decide to proceed in the search process for a new system, the third step is the evaluation and selection of the software application. In the traditional software evaluation process, an organization looks at all major vendors that meet the identified functional specifications and rates each with some type of scorecard. As an alternative, I recommend a "proof-of-concept" where you use experts (e.g. accounting or auditing firm or industry IS consultants) to do a first pass of vendor products and develop a list of two or three top candidates. These candidates (and their resellers or certified vendors) should then be evaluated in several core areas:

- Ability to meet your organization's core functional specifications
- Customer references regarding system functionality, implementation and training, and service and support
- Ability to interface with your practice management, MCO, and or other software applications for analysis and reporting
- Report writer capabilities
- Financial stability
- Price

Once a vendor has been selected and a contract negotiated and signed, the final step is to plan a successful implementation.

Ensuring Implementation Success

While all software implementations require good planning and project management skills, the unique nature of implementing a new financial management information system demands some special tips for success:

- Don't wait until your fiscal year changes

- When building an implementation team, put permanent staff on the new system and have any temporary staff maintain the old system
- Re-engineer as you implement
- Get the set-up right from the start
- Remember that reports are what it is all about

Don't Wait Until Your Fiscal Year Changes

When implementing new financial management information systems, many CFOs and finance departments insist on making the change coincide with a change in the organization's fiscal year. However, doing so can pose its own challenges and problems. You are severely limited in your options for when you start using the system and in making changes in the implementation plan as needed. (Changing at a fiscal year tends to force an "all or nothing" switchover on the first day of the fiscal year.) And, core implementation tasks occur simultaneously with fiscal year-end responsibilities, and finance staff are heavily involved in both sets of activities.

Given that you are likely to run "dual" systems for a period of time, it is actually easier to plan to go-live with the new system during a month that is not a fiscal year change. A good plan will balance the ease of implementation with a quick release of major functionality.

When Building an Implementation Team, Put Permanent Staff on the New System and Have Any Temporary Staff Maintain the Old System

The key here is to dedicate your best and most knowledgeable finance staff to plan and execute the implementation of the new financial management system. Use temporary staff as needed for routine finance functions on the old system. As with all software conversions, the implementation team's responsibilities should include system planning and set-up, data conversion, testing, and training.

Reengineer as You Implement

Make certain that you re-engineer your fiscal processes (e.g., workflow and paperwork for accounts payable and payroll, month-end reporting processes, etc.) during implementation to take best advantage of the system's capabilities.

Get the Set-Up Right From the Start

Probably the most crucial part of implementing a new financial management information system is getting the configuration tables set up optimally from the beginning. These tables, particularly the chart of accounts, drive most of the reporting and analysis functions of the system, so it is important to use the system change as a time to re-think how you structure and report financial information. (E.g., do you need to re-arrange the chart of accounts for better product line financial reporting or to do activity-based cost management?)

Remember That Reports Are What It Is All About

The system implementation must include plans for releasing required financial and management analysis reports right from the start. Make certain that your team focuses heavily on designing and implementing usage of these reports, and dedicate extensive time to training staff to read and use the management information that they contain. In cases where the reports generate information from data that is imported from other systems (or data-warehoused as needed) be certain that the integrity of the data is assured and that clear timetables have been established for the frequency of integrating the data based upon management needs. ◨

Marketing & Development

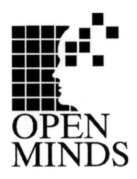

OPEN
MINDS

Strategic Positioning & Strategic Planning: Integrating Critical Marketing, Operations & Finance Functions for Success

Joseph P. Naughton-Travers, Ed.M.

In today's behavioral health and social service market, few provider organizations have developed formal marketing functions, and fewer still have integrated marketing operations and financial planning. Yet, in turbulent and changing times, success for these organizations will be based on how well they can strategically "position" themselves against the competition.

What is strategic positioning? — It is the inclusion of market positioning as a key objective in the strategic business planning process.

Chances are that you already have a formal strategic planning process at your organization. It involves clarifying your organization's mission and objectives, assessing the external environment and your internal capabilities, and then building a plan to deploy your staff and resources to achieve your mission.

But, the strategic plans of many organizations in our field are missing one key ingredient — inclusion of market positioning and other strategies and tactics needed for success in a competitive market. In years past, when the behavioral health and social service field was highly- regulated and resources were allocated without direct competition, market positioning was irrelevant. But all that has changed in the past few years.

Positioning is a marketing term for how to manage the "marketing mix" relative to the competition in order to maximize the appeal of your organization and its services to target customers. In marketing management, organizations can only control four organizational attributes (known in marketing theory as the four "P"s):

- Product — What services do our customers want? What "performance" and "value" attributes do customers want?
- Price — What price are customers willing to pay for these services and for specific levels of performance?
- Promotion — How do we communicate the value and features of our services to customers and others who influence our customers?
- Place — How do we contract for our services? How do customers select our services?

The goal of market positioning is two-fold:
- To create real differentiation between our organization and our competitors
- To make the differences known to our customers

The key issue with market positioning is the relative value of your organization's services in the minds of customers — a careful balance between quality and cost.

In this article, we discuss the important roles that marketing, operational, and financial planning all play in the strategic positioning process.

As is typical in historical strategic planning, a thorough understanding of the environment and a critical analysis of internal functionality are key. However, a competitive marketplace introduces new factors — market segmentation by customer type; market differentiation in comparison to competitors; market positioning relative to competition; and target costing. The roles of these considerations in the strategic planning process are illustrated in the accompanying chart in figure 1.

The Role of Marketing in Strategic Positioning & Strategic Planning

Your organization's marketing department is responsible for three elements of the strategic positioning process — the market analysis, the competitor analysis, and later, the marketing promotion and tactics plan. The market analysis should be an on-going data collection process designed to answer several key questions:

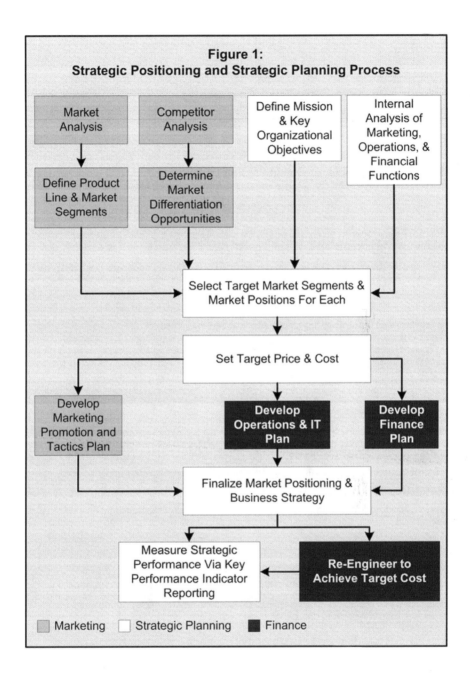

Figure 1:
Strategic Positioning and Strategic Planning Process

Who Are Our Customers, and What Do They Want?

The goal here it to not only have a clear understanding of your customer demographics (both purchasers and consumers) but to know how they perceive your organization (image assessment), how they define value and quality, and what services they really want.

How Much Are Customers Willing to Pay for Services?

Unfortunately, price remains the primary selection criteria in today's predominantly undifferentiated behavioral health and social service market. While your long-term marketing plan will likely include efforts to shift the customer focus from price to "value," it is critical that you have a clear sense of the acceptable price points for services in order develop a positioning strategy.

What Trends Are Influencing the Market at This Time?

Here you are looking for major market trends, such as shifts in financing, service delivery system structure, legislation, and consumer and provider movements, which will require changes in your organization's strategic plan.

The second element of the strategic positioning process completed by your marketing department is the competitor analysis. Here the task is to gather information about who your competitors are for each service line (including market share information), how they are perceived by customers (better or worse than your organization and why), and how much they charge for services.

Once you've completed both the market and competitor analyses, the next steps are to:

- Define your product line and analyze the segments of the customer market — Segmentation is the process of aggregating customers with similar wants and values into groups. Segmentation can be done on a variety of demographic, geographic, and psychological factors, and is used to develop a marketing strategy specific to selected target market segments.
- Determine differentiation opportunities from competitors — Here the task is to identify ways that your market positioning strategy can set your

organization apart from competitors based upon factors customers care about.

Ensuring Business Planning Is Truly Strategic

The strategic planning function of your organization has the responsibility of clarifying the organization's mission and objectives, completing an analysis of internal capabilities, and then integrating these with the market and competitor data and analyses compiled by the marketing department. Next, the planning process moves on to select target customer segments, develop a positioning strategy for each of them, and then to build the operations, IT, and finance workplans to support the strategic plan. Once target customers and market positions are selected, your marketing staff can then develop their promotion and tactics plan.

The challenge at this juncture is to make certain that your planning processes are really strategic. For many organizations, strategic planning has become perfunctory and ritualistic, akin to updating last year's budget and then putting it back on the shelf. Your organization's missions should be clear and meaningful, and the plan must have actionable objectives. The process must include a frank assessment of your organization's strengths and weaknesses and should incorporate the up-to-date market and competitor data and analyses discussed in the previous section.

There are six primary positioning strategies for behavioral health and social services providers:

- Low Cost Position — This is the "Walmart" strategy — marketing your organization as the one with the lowest price. Most providers are trying to escape this position where the competitive strategy is based solely on price.
- High Cost and High Value Position — This is the "Ritz Carlton" approach. "We offer the highest quality services for discriminating customers." It is the market position everyone wants, but few get to have.
- Best Value Position — This position strives to find a balance between the low-cost and high-cost positions by focusing on how target customers define quality and value, then building services based upon these at a "reasonable" price.

- High Tech Position — This strategy is newer in behavioral health and social services and strives to position your organization as the one with using the "latest and greatest" technology. Examples might include promoting the use of Internet-based services and computer-assisted treatment planning.
- The Integrated Position — This is the continuum of care strategy. "We are part of a integrated network that can coordinate your care from one level of service to another."
- Niche Position — This strategy attempts to differentiate an organization from competitors based on specialty services in demand by customers (e.g., providing foster homes for adolescent sex offenders) or on specific product features (such as offering weekend services or convenient locations).

Making Finance Strategic With Target Costing

A critical component of the finance plan and your positioning strategy is the target price for your services. In order to develop a successful market position, your organization must incorporate strategic cost management principles into its business planning process. Essentially, this means moving towards market-driven costing and pricing based upon the data collected in your market and competitor analyses. There are three types of costs:

- Planned Costs: These are the costs assumed for delivering a service in a particular time period — essentially the traditional "budgeted" costs.
- Actual Costs: These are the actual costs incurred when delivering a service.
- Target Costs: These are the costs you aim to achieve, based upon customer demands and competitive market pressures.

Simply put, the target cost is a competitive price minus the desired profit. Thus, the concept of target costing is essentially a "top-to-bottom" approach to pricing and delivering services, where you first determine a competitive price, then figure out how to re-engineer your operations to achieve it. It requires careful coordination between your organization's marketing, operations, and finance functions.

The first step in target costing uses your marketing data — clear and up-to-date information about what customers want, how much they are willing to pay, and what competitors charge for services. You set a target price for the service based upon your positioning strategy, along with a desired profit margin. This produces the target cost for the service. Your finance department then has the challenge of determining and managing unit costs in order to achieve the target cost for the service. Most commonly, this is accomplished by using activity-based cost management principles to report the cost components of services, to eliminate non-essential components, and to implement process improvements to reduce unit costs.

Thus, target costing is both strategic and operational — strategic in the sense that costs are linked to competitive prices, and operational in that target costs are reached by carefully managing and re-engineering operations. (See figure 2.)

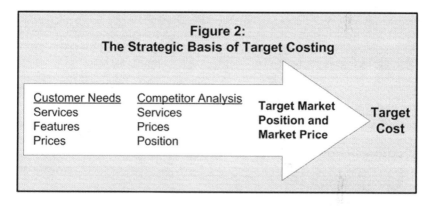

Figure 2:
The Strategic Basis of Target Costing

Now that you've identified your target market segments and their market positions and set target prices and costs for your services, you are ready to build the marketing, operations, IT, and finance workplans to realize your strategic plan and market position.

Achieving Your Goals: Measuring Strategic Performance

The last step in the strategic positioning process is to make certain that you and your managers know whether or not the strategic objectives and market position are being achieved. This is accomplished by building a key performance measurement (KPI) system to report progress. An effective performance measurement system uses financial and non-financial measures and is driven by structured data from the information system. The KPIs represent those data points that measure the "health" of your organization in five major categories:

- Financial — These measures reflect the overall financial status for your organization and should include comparisons of actual costs to the target costs for services.

- Customer — These measures reflect customer satisfaction (from both consumers and purchasers), image assessment (i.e., was our positioning and promotion strategy effective?), and whether or not the target market share was achieved.

- Innovation — These measures reflect your organization's commitment to acquiring and implementing new knowledge.

- Internal — These measures reflect the overall health of your organization's internal operations.

- Progress Toward Strategic Actions — These measures report the progress of critical tasks and strategic actions based upon the timelines you set during your planning process.

Ideally, performance measures are reported on a monthly basis, with data for the current month as well as the previous 12 months to assist your staff in identifying trends in performance and instituting corrective actions when things don't go according to plan! ▧

Moving to a "Customer-Driven" Competitive Strategy: The Information & Analysis Needed for Strategic Market Positioning

Monica E. Oss, M.S.

Ask most professionals and managers in the behavioral health and social service field if their organization is "customer driven" and the most frequent answer is "yes." However, I've found that most organizations are customer driven in concept, but not in practice. The fundamental problem is that the executive teams of most organizations in the field have not developed a marketing infrastructure to gather and analyze the customer data needed for competitive positioning of their services.

Admittedly, there are some complex factors that are impediments to moving organizations to a customer-driven management orientation. There are regulatory impediments that interfere with delivering truly consumer-driven services. Rules about licensure, accreditation, and benefit plan design create the boundaries for service system evolution. Some financing and reimbursement models, both historical program-specific models and restrictive managed care models, limit flexibility and interfere with the delivery of consumer-centric services. (And, in some states and counties, current policy penalizes more customer-oriented organizations.) These factors are characteristics of the structure of our "industry" and are only half of the strategic positioning equation. The other half of the equation is competitive positioning — the value (when comparing price and benefits) that an organization offers its customers when compared to its competitors. (For an extensive discussion of industry structure and relative competitive positioning, refer to the work of Michael Porter.)

Since most organizations wouldn't consider altering their missions and leaving the field, there are only two directions for strategy. The first is to use advocacy and political organizing to shape the policies that affect the structure of the field. The second is to develop strategies to achieve more favorable organizational positioning in the context of those changes in the field. Fundamentally, there are only two sustainable market positions in any field — low cost positioning and positioning on service differentiation. The lack of a customer-driven orientation and related management practices has, by default, resulted in commodity pricing becoming the standard. As the consolidation of purchasing power (through managed care and privatization) and the pressures of supply and demand have dropped "market" rates, the cost/price threshold has dropped.

Coping with the financial effects of this commodity-pricing phenomenon, and the need to adopt more customer-driven planning models for the purposes of differentiation, are the strategic factors facing most executive teams today. The key planning questions are:

- How does an organization increase its operational efficiencies and reduce costs enough to "survive" the current wave of commodity pricing?
- How do executive teams reposition their services as "differentiated" in order to move out of competition based on low price?

For most organizations, these two solutions need to happen simultaneously and quickly. On the "survival" issue, the advice is relatively simple — know and track unit costs and eliminate expenses for activities that are not valued by the customers. With regard to repositioning and market-driven service differentiation, the primary issue is whether or not the current services that your organization provides have a "value" to customers that exceeds the "value" offered by the competition. This involves an analytical process of understanding your customers well enough to make those judgments and then acting on that understanding.

The likely results of gaining this organizational understanding of market factors are the investment in services that have clear customer value and preference; the elimination of high-cost (compared to competitors) services from the "service mix" that do not have the potential for differentiation on an attribute other than price; and the clear occupancy of the "low price" niche in the remainder. At the point those strategic decisions are made, marketing becomes the critical factor — successful "market differentiation" requires a marketing plan that recognizes customer preferences through product differentiation, pricing strategies, cooperative distribution agreements, and promotion.

There are four key types of information that are critical to assessing competitive advantage and developing a positioning strategy:

- Customer Profiling
- Product Line and Portfolio Analysis
- Environmental and Market Trend Analysis
- Competitor Profiling

Step 1: Creating Customer Profiles

First and foremost, it is important to understand both who your customers are and what they want. Behavioral health and social service organizations have two sets of customers — purchasers and service consumers. It is important to clarify how their values and expectations both differ and overlap. Preliminary customer profiling and analysis should include customer demographic segmentation, consumer and payer "value" analysis (service preferences in terms of benefits and costs), and customer image assessment (customer perceptions of your organization's value relative to competitors).

Step 2: Product Line & Portfolio Analysis

Once you have a better understanding of both sets of your customers, the next step is to begin a formal analysis of your product lines (programs and services), individually and in their entirety (the entire portfolio). The first step is to clearly define what services your organization offers, key benefits offered, what consumer populations they target, payment sources for those services, and how they fit into an overall continuum of service offerings within your organization.

With your services defined, you can then move on to review their performance, cost, and profitability. You need to answer such questions as — What is the total cost of each program (including allocation of overhead)? What is the unit cost of services, as well as the cost of a typical service episode? How do these unit costs compare with those of your competitors and with industry standards? How effective are programs and services in meeting their customer- defined performance objectives? What services result in the best outcomes from the customers' perspectives? For what services do expenses exceed revenues? And, if you are a non-profit organization, how are charitable resources allocated among product lines?

When completing your product line analysis, it is important to revisit your costing and pricing methodology. Are overhead expenses allocated based on revenue, employees, or number of consumers? Is your service pricing by the program, by the unit, by the case, in bundled rates, capitated, and/or performance-based? Do you offer services using pricing models that are attractive to purchasers?

Step 3: Analyzing Overall Market Trends

In order to develop strategies for responding to changes in the structure of the field, competitive pressures, and changing customer preferences, an understanding of the external environment is essential. What is the total market (in terms of consumers, dollars spent, number of payers, etc.) for each service? What market share does the service have? Are the total market and your organization's market share increasing or decreasing? What are the major trends in the financing and service delivery structure system, and how will they effect your organization? Is there new legislation or pending actions by federal, state, or local organizations that could affect the market? Are there consumer advocacy movements pushing for policy changes in the service delivery system?

Step 4: Sizing Up Competitors

The last major information set required for this strategic planning process is competitor profiles. Once you've developed a preliminary list of competitors for each service, the next step is to gather data that will assist you in your understanding of your current strategic positioning. What services do competitors offer and how do they price them? How do customers perceive your competitors in terms of price, features, and quality? How do competitors promote their services, and what is their apparent market strategy?

The information gathering process is not as daunting as it might first appear. Some customer profiling information should be available from your own management information system (MIS). In addition, census data, published reports, and web sites can fill in many blanks. Information specific to customers' perceptions of service value are always externally gathered (usually by surveys, informational interviews, focus groups, etc.). The product line analysis can typically be developed as an executive team exercise in order to clarify service descriptions, operating processes, and organizational objectives. A financial analysis is also necessary to determine program costs and unit costs. While most executives are already aware of major market trends, estimates of consumer demand, reimbursement types and amounts, and other quantitative information usually requires additional data gathering from published sources or from primary research. Competitor data can be gathered from promotional materials, web sites, industry publications, professional associations, telephone calls to other executives, and reports to regulatory organizations.

Using Customer Information to Develop a Competitive Strategy

Once all the research has been completed, how do you use it to develop a plan of action? The focused data gathering process gives you a clear understanding of who your customers are, what they want, your competitors, and how your services "fit" into the market. Can your organization develop a competitive advantage based on low cost for any of its services? If not, the key is to use the information gathered to determine how to set your organization apart from the rest of the pack. For example, can you differentiate by targeting services to specific consumer segments or in specific geographic areas? Should you develop specialized services for a critical consumer population? Can you implement a pricing strategy unique to your market that is more attractive to purchasers? Can you demonstrate better performance and/or outcomes than your competitors?

So how does this notion of the customer-driven organization address the commodity pricing phenomenon in the field? Customer-centered organizations have the orientation and the infrastructure to gather and use market information to continually differentiate themselves from their competitors and remain successful in the market. This process enables executive teams to make wise resource allocation decisions, such as when to subsidize services; in which services to invest additional development resources; and how to focus advocacy activities.

You may believe that the health and human service field can never be truly consumer driven; that these services are too technical and too complex for the average person to know what they want; that public agency missions can never (or should never) be driven by market forces. Philosophically, this may be correct. Practically, it is a dangerous assumption for many organizations in the field. If we fail to understand what our customers value, we run the risk of having consumers and payers bypass the traditional service sector and select other alternatives for problem resolution. Moving forward, successful organizations will have a customer-driven management framework where poor-performing programs (as defined by our customers, our missions, and our strategic objectives) are eliminated; where good programs are made better, and great programs are given the resources to grow and evolve. ▣

Marketing & Development Competency

Issues in Access to New Treatment Options for Individuals With Severe Depression

Monica E. Oss, M.S. & J. Jay Mackie, Ph.D.

A wide range of new technologies will soon be available to consumers to address mental health, neurological health, and intellectual disability problems. Even as emerging therapies are made accessible to consumers, it is likely that these new treatments will not have the maximum clinical or financial impact on health conditions due to several potential obstacles. One such obstacle is the absence of standardized payer policies in place to address the appropriateness of new technologies, an issue that needs to be considered sooner than later. Additionally, challenges regarding adaptation of these new technologies to clinical and administrative management structures need to be reviewed...

Depression Treatment Efficacy — Research Implications for Treatment Guidelines

Researchers have studied depression and its related treatment for decades. The most recent research was conducted by the National Institute of Mental Health (NIMH). The Sequenced Treatment Alternatives to Relieve Depression (STAR*D) Study2[1] has provided the health care community with new perspectives on the effectiveness of currently available treatment options for depression. STAR*D was a seven-year, 4,000-consumer study to determine the best "next-step" treatments for patients failing to respond to prior treatment attempts. STAR*D was also designed to compare relative efficacy of different treatment strategies and specific treatments; and to provide important information on the long-term course of depression, including its nature and the timing of relapses.

---

1 Trivedi, M., Rush, A.J., et. al. (2006, January). Evaluation of outcomes with citalopram for depression using measurement-based care in STAR-D: Implications for clinical practice. *American Journal of Psychiatry*, 163:28-40.

The STAR*D research findings are numerous and compelling. One critical finding for health care policy is that after using four different courses of currently available treatment options, only 67% of patients achieved remission of their symptoms. The Task Force members discussed the implications of this finding on policy and practice. It is clear that no one medication (or combinations of medications and/or cognitive therapies) is a panacea for all consumers and the clinical predictors of treatment selection are weak. In addition, current depression treatment guidelines are limited in their utility for addressing the needs of all consumers with depression. Current guidelines address the use of medication and cognitive behavioral therapy (CBT) in a process involving selection of initial medication use and subsequent combination therapies. These guidelines assume that remission of symptoms is achieved. However, the current guidelines do not address interventions for the 33% of consumers who do not achieve remission of their depression using currently available therapies. These consumers have a level of disease known as treatment-resistant depression.

Indeed, this severity of illness in depression must be recognized and needs to be incorporated into the existing treatment guidelines. Also needed is the creation of a methodology for identifying consumers with treatment-resistant depression. Within the scientific community, the current definition ranges from two to four failed treatments.[2]

The lack of a standardized definition creates problems for consumers, clinicians, and payers. Without consensus regarding appropriate treatment algorithms, it is difficult to determine the related costs or to evaluate the appropriateness of new treatment methodologies for consumers of different clinical profiles.

Health Care Related Costs of Treatment-Resistant Depression

The cost of depression in the United States in the year 2000 was estimated to be $83 billion. Of this figure, $26 billion was associated with treatment costs and

---

2 Rush, A. J., Trivedi, M.et al. (2006, November). Acute and longer-term outcomes in depressed outpatients requiring one or several treatment steps: a STAR*D report. *American Journal of Psychiatry*, 163 (11): 1905-17.

the remaining $57 billion in costs was due to absenteeism, reduced productivity at work, and the value of lifetime earnings lost as a result of suicide-related deaths.[3] While the costs of depression are certainly significant, the major portion of costs can be attributed to the condition of treatment-resistant depression. A recent study found that the annual treatment costs for individuals with non-treatment-resistant depression were $6,500 while the annual costs for individuals with treatment-resistant depression were over six times that amount, or $42,300.[4] (In this study, individuals with treatment-resistant depression were defined as those who switched medications at least once, were hospitalized, and/or had a recorded suicide attempt.) Another study found that total health care costs for individuals with treatment-resistant depression (defined as eight medication switches) were $14,000 versus $6,200 for those with two medication switches or less.[5] For those organizations that provide health care benefits, whether corporations, government entities, or health plans, treatment-resistant depression is a major cost contributor.

From an ethical and moral standpoint, in addition to being arguably more important than the issues surrounding health care costs associated with chronic depression, one must consider the issue of suicide. In 2001, in the United States, suicide took the lives of 30,622 people; 132,353 individuals were hospitalized following suicide attempts; and 116,639 were treated in emergency departments and released.[6] Depression is a major risk factor for suicide and individuals whose depressive symptoms are not relieved through conventional treatment are at elevated risk for suicide.

3 Questions and answers about the NIMH sequenced treatment alternatives to relieve depression (STAR*D) study — background. (2006, January). Retrieved February 1, 2007, from National Institute on Mental Health Web site: http://www.nimh.nih.gov/healthinformation/stard_qa_general.cfm

4 Crown, W.H., Finkelstein, S., Berndt, E.R., et. al. (2002). The impact of treatment-resistant depression on health care utilization and costs. *Journal of Clinical Psychiatry*, 63: 963 – 971.

5 Russell, J.M., Hawkins, K., Ozminkowski, R.J., et al. (2004). The cost consequences of treatment-resistant depression. *Journal of Clinical Psychiatry*, 65: 341 – 347.

6 Suicide Fact Sheet. (2006, September 7). Retrieved February 1, 2007 from the National Center for Injury Prevention & Control Web Site: http://www.cdc.gov/ncipc/factsheets/suifacts.htm

Standards of Scientific Evidence and Consumer Access to New Technologies

Given the limited efficacy of currently available treatments for a third of the consumer population with depression, and the costs of treatment-resistant consumers to health plans, the question of treatment alternatives arises. There is an emerging group of nonpharmaceutical neurotechnology treatments for consideration in patient care. There are two related questions to contemplate as health care payers and policymakers evaluate the issues of evidence required to make decisions to facilitate consumer access to these emerging neurotechnologies. The first is a question relevant to all chronic health care conditions — what evidence and related policies are required to determine that a new treatment is safe and/or efficacious for individuals with chronic health care conditions? The second question is one of treatment options — how should this evidence be evaluated in situations where consumers have a life-threatening disease and no other treatment options?

With regard to evaluation of treatments for chronic disease, there has been discussion of alternatives to the use of randomized controlled trials (RCT). RCT has long been the 'gold standard' of evidence for approval by the Food and Drug Administration (FDA).

However, RCT has limitations in the evaluation of treatment interventions for chronic diseases. RCT designs are typically short-term, consider a single variable, and do not evaluate efficacy in the context of complex, multi-factor chronic diseases. In fact, RCT study designs typically exclude individuals with chronic illness because of design requirements to withhold treatment from a 'control' group — a clinical situation that is neither practical nor ethical for individuals with a chronic life-threatening disease.[7]

As the scientific and regulatory community considers the effectiveness of emerging treatments for chronic disease, research design should move beyond RCT. STAR*D is one such example —a "practical trial" that assessed

---

7 Menza, M. (2006, July). STAR-D: The results begin to roll in. *American Journal of Psychiatry*, 163:7.

effectiveness in real-world clinical situations[8] Another such methodological option is the practice-based evidence (PBE) study design.[9] PBE is a prospective, observational, cohort study methodology that allows analysis of 'real world' treatment factors (interventions, processes, professionals, etc.) and consumer factors (diagnoses, functionality, demographic characteristics, etc.) over time. These types of approaches can employ severity adjustment methodologies to remove selection bias, a critical factor for evaluating chronic conditions, and have the benefit of comparing active treatments in terms of a number of clinical outcomes. Research approaches like practical trials and PBE are better suited to evaluate new treatments for chronic diseases than traditional RCT models.

For consumers, payers, and regulators, the juxtaposition of limited treatment options, costs of the illness, and ill-fitting standards of evidence have created a 'perfect policy storm.' A third of consumers suffering from depression do not respond to available treatment options and are at high risk for increased illness and mortality at a significant cost to health plans. At the same time, the standards of evidence typically used to assess new health care interventions are not appropriate in a population with a chronic condition like depression.

To resolve this situation, the health care field needs a collaborative industry initiative — representing regulators, payers, and consumers — to develop a shared set of standards for addressing the issues of policy, financing, and practice for these emerging neurotechnologies. For each emerging treatment intervention, a collaborative consensus is needed to specify the instances where conditional use should be permitted and to establish shared clinical criteria for conditional use. In addition, a collaborative consensus is needed on standards of evidence for chronic health care conditions and a scientifically valid model for measuring the efficacy of each intervention in the population that is granted conditional use to the new treatment intervention.

In the near future, the fruits of extensive clinical research will yield an expanding array of new neurotechnologies that will be available to consumers. These new technologies enter a health care policy environment where the

---

8 Insel,T. (2006, January). Beyond efficacy: The STAR-D trial. *American Journal of Psychiatry*, 163:1

9 Horn, S. (2006, June). Alternative methods for practice-based evidence. (Annual Research Meeting 2006 PowerPoint Presentation) Seattle, Washington.

standards of evidence must be reevaluated to address the growing proportion of health care conditions that are chronic rather than acute. This evaluation must also consider the rapid growth in health care spending on these chronic conditions. To address this situation, payers need new clinical guidelines and standards of evidence to assure appropriate use of health care resources and safety for their members. These guidelines and standards must be forged by a consensus with regulators and consumer advocates. At the same time, these new standards must provide consumers who suffer from life-threatening conditions, and no other treatment options, with timely and appropriate access to these new treatment alternatives. ▣

Information Technology

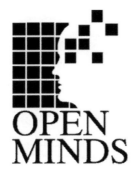

OPEN
MINDS

A Forward Look: How New Technologies Are Changing the Field

Monica E. Oss, M.S.

We don't often think of the behavioral health and disability supports field as a "technology rich" environment, but the fact is that new technological developments in biotechnology, computing, telecommunications, genetics, and other fields are ushering in a new era of opportunity and challenge. What is the link between these new technologies, the theory of "disruptive innovations," and the day-to-day business activities of behavioral health organizations? What specific disruptive effect will all these changes really have on the field? The adoption of new technologies will alter the field in five distinct areas:

1. More self-service by consumers
2. Highly trained professionals working only on most complex cases
3. More home-based services, with a corresponding decrease in use of high-intensity institutions
4. The natural tendency to integrate services from a variety of sources
5. The "offshoring" effect

More Self-Service

In every aspect of life and business, we see an obvious trend toward consumers doing more for themselves. We manage our own banking needs on-line and through ATM machines; we book our own travel on-line as well, as opposed to the "old" technology of using a travel agent. We pump our own gasoline, and check ourselves out at the grocery store. The behavioral health and disability services fields are no different. Any technology that allows consumers to do more for themselves — such as on-line diagnostic tools and remote monitoring programs — will be adopted by consumers because they are less expensive and provide more control and convenience. Consumers are taking control and engaging with "self-serve" technologies across the field. On-line treatment programs, such as MoodGYM and eGetgoing, are taking the field by storm. New programs that provide professional consultation via e-mail (such as Ask-the-Internet- Therapist), as well as video and virtual reality applications for behavioral and cognitive disorders — such as Fearfighter and Calipso — are already on the market. As consumers do more for themselves, they need you (service provider organizations and professionals) less. And health plans and other payers will pay for these technologies because they are less costly.

Highly Specialized Professionals for Only the Most Complex Cases

Even with the self-service phenomenon, there will always be some things that consumers cannot do for themselves — like prescribing their own medications. But new technologies will replace some functions so that the same level of specialization and training will not be needed as in the past. For instance, as new psychotropic medications become safer, primary care physicians, rather than psychiatrists, are more willing to prescribe and manage them. This decreases the need for more highly trained psychiatrists in favor of "generalist" professionals.

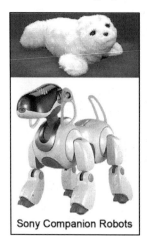

Sony Companion Robots

The United Kingdom's National Health Service is using CD-ROM-based, self-directed treatment for mild and moderate depression. Expert system-based technologies decrease the need for mental health professionals for consumers, focusing their work on individuals with the most severe and treatment-resistant depression.

In disability supports, medical monitors will collect indicators of the health status of an individual 24 hours a day through wearable consumer tracking technologies that monitor blood pressure, heart rate, blood glucose levels, and skin temperature — and transmit that information to a central monitoring center. Intelligence and judgment functions will be automated and managed remotely. The result will be that highly trained professionals such as registered nurses, who once did the gathering of medical indicators, will ultimately be replaced with (or become) less specialized (and lower-cost) workers, such as home health care aides. The role of the nurse will be limited to interventions with those patients having "outlier" medical indicators.

Across the board, technologies that support the use of less time of highly trained professionals will gain rapid acceptance. The challenge for service organizations is repositioning their core competencies around the consumer with "complex" conditions and requirements.

More Home-Based Services

Many of the new technologies that are changing the field are designed to enable consumers of all kinds to stay in their homes. In-home supports, such as QuietCare by Ecumen, and other technologies help to identify small health issues before they become larger. QuietCare is an early detection/warning system that provides caregivers with round-the-clock information and alerts about the safety and well-being of elderly or other at-risk individuals, while maintaining their privacy and independence. The system uses discreet wireless activity sensors that are positioned throughout a residence to learn his/her normal pattern of daily living such as meal preparation, interaction with medications and bathroom use, as well as morning wake-up time and overall activity. The system remotely identifies potential medical emergencies, such as possible bathroom falls, and automatically alerts caregivers to these situations, thereby permitting them to provide early intervention.

The Gesture Pendant project is another such technology, created through a collaboration between the College of Computing's Contextual Computing Group and the Interactive Media Technology Center. The Gesture Pendant allows ordinary household devices to be controlled, literally, with the wave of a hand. The user wears

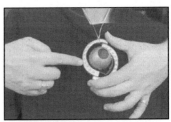
Gesture Pendant from Georgia Institute of Technology

a small pendant that contains a wireless camera. The user makes gestures in front of the pendant that controls household appliances using simple hand gestures. The pendant system can also analyze the user's movement as he/she makes gestures, looking for loss of motor skill or tremors that might indicate the onset of illness or problems with medication. It can also observe daily activities to determine, for example, if a person has been eating regularly and moving around. This monitoring provides an aid for elderly or disabled persons, because it requires less dexterity, memory, and eyesight than traditional remote controls and therefore helps users achieve more independence in their homes.

Through technologies like these, people who previously couldn't stay at home now have the option to "age in place" or remain in community settings. Home-based services are already having a significant impact on the number of people in more intense institutional settings.

The Natural Tendency to "Integrate"

In times gone by, when consumers needed a specialist, they worked with a variety of disparate and disconnected professionals and organizations — everything from the hospital neurology department, community mental health professionals, to service agencies for mental retardation or child protection and welfare. New technologies are going to intermingle services from all these "silos" — so that, for example, a person with co-occurring mental and substance use disorders, low IQ, and diabetes will no longer need four case managers to address their needs and organize services. Ultimately, such a person will go to their primary care physician (or "medical home") for care management, and access specialists as needed. Changes in technology will speed the integration process, "scrambling" services from a variety of provider sources. Provider organizations and professionals in specialties such as behavioral health will need to develop models to integrate across complex consumer needs.

The Offshoring Effect

Last, but not least, the behavioral health and disabilities support fields are subject to the "offshoring effect" (the relocation of services or jobs elsewhere in order to reduce costs). And the physical location of off-shored services matters very little. India or Indiana, the key factor is the payer's perception of quality and cost — and acceptance of the technology that makes it happen.

Some specific services in the field are highly and imminently "off-shorable," including:
1. All talking therapies
2. Medical and health education of both professionals and consumers
3. All types of consumer and family support programs
4. Monitoring of home-bound and institutionalized individuals, including foster homes
5. Medical and health status evaluations

6. Psychological testing
7. Service algorithm management

Traditional in-person services are already being replaced with suicide and mental health hotlines — staffed from overseas locations — and by an increasingly diverse variety of remote and computer-based psychotherapy tools and services. For consumers, more options, more control, and more convenience make this a no-brainer. For payers, the question is simple: Can I get a service of the same value for less money? In most cases, the answer will be yes. For provider organizations and professionals, this creates a two-edged strategic sword:

- Can our traditional services hold up to a comparison of consumer quality and lower payer costs?
- Can our organization move services offshore to other jurisdictions, using technology?

Without a doubt, these functional components — and probably many more to come — of behavioral health and social services can, and will, be off-shored either within or outside of the United States.

So Who Can Survive?

The disruption of business-as-usual caused by emerging technologies is a daunting prospect for many organizations in the field. We are poised for a "perfect storm" of macro-market factors, with payers pushing new strategies and new technologies because they are less expensive, and consumers pulling for them because they want the added convenience and control that they provide.

So how can professionals and provider organizations, with limited resources, weather the storm? The answer is in keeping the consumer "problem" and consumer demand in focus, and becoming an expert on solutions (rather than a specific process). Remember that the number of people receiving behavioral health and disability treatment and support is increasing, and so are the assistive technologies and options available to serve them.

The "market-focused" organization won't be resistant to learning about all of the options available to consumers. These organizations will be most successful through this period of rapid change and will develop a number of key characteristics:

- Ability to operate within integrated systems (as defined by the local market)
- Capacity to accept risk-based or performance-based reimbursement (as defined by the payer)
- Consumer-centric services (as defined by local consumer characteristics)
- Ability to demonstrate a value-proposition that resonates with both payers and consumers
- Systems in place to deliver as much service in home-based environments as technologically feasible and preferred by consumers

You can decide for yourself about whether particular technologies or products are good or bad, but you can't ignore that they exist — and that they are here now. Having the knowledge and judgment to advise consumers on the relative benefits of new technologies and service offerings is the definition of a new category of professional: The Solutions Expert. ▩

Strategic Leverage Through Technology in Behavioral Health & Social Service Organizations: Key Is Integrating Technology Planning With Organizational Strategy

Joseph P. Naughton-Travers, Ed.M.

The role that technology can play in behavioral health and social service organizations is multi- faceted. It can allow rapid access to consumer demographic, clinical, and service information across an organization. Software applications can automate repetitive tasks, provide critical performance data, ensure consistency in service planning, and monitor quality and outcomes. Communication can be enhanced with video conferencing, e-mail, internet access, and state-of- the-art telephone systems. Access to data and software applications has been made easier with wireless devices and application service providers.

With so much technology now available to the field — from traditional practice management and managed care software applications to the latest in Internet and wireless capabilities — how does an organization get the maximum leverage for its technology investments? What is "best practice" in planning and budgeting for technology? Historically, organizations in the behavioral health and social service field have been slow to purchase technology, and for many organizations, implementing core technologies (such as practice management systems) has been bumpy at best and disastrous at worst. Yet today's competitive marketplace does not allow for wasted financial and management resources, and misdirected or ineffective technology spending is too costly for most organizations.

The key to successful technology planning is to integrate it with your organization's strategic planning and budgeting process. The goal is not to use technology simply because it exists, but rather to use only the technology that your organization needs to achieve its key strategic and operational objectives. This could mean that you can get by without the latest upgrade to your major software applications, or it may mean that you need to make considerable investment in the latest technology. In this article, we describe a recommended strategic technology planning process as well as address the common questions that arise for organizations when doing their technology planning.

Strategic Technology Planning

What is strategic technology planning? Essentially, it is the process of identifying the technological infrastructure necessary for your organization to achieve its strategic and operational objectives. What critical business functionality does your organization need from software applications in order to meet its objectives? Can technological advances in telecommunications, the Internet, and wireless technology play a major role in improving your organizational performance, reducing operating costs, or increasing stakeholder satisfaction and preference in your organization?

By integrating technology planning with your strategic planning and budgeting process, you ensure that technology planning no longer occurs in a vacuum. Rather, like all budget items, technology planning becomes a strategic resource allocation decision — which technology investments are necessary and which are not?

There are three common questions that come up for behavioral health and social service organizations when they are developing their technology strategies:
1. How do we decide what technology we need?
2. How much should we be spending on technology?
3. Should we buy or build the technology we need?

Let's review these three questions briefly before laying out the step-by-step process for strategic technology planning.

1. How Do We Decide What Technology We Need?

The first issue many behavioral health and social service organizations wrestle with is figuring out what technologies they need — and probably equally importantly, which ones they don't. This is often the result of a poorly constructed or poorly communicated strategic plan. A good strategic business plan clarifies the organizational mission and vision, and then develops clear strategic objectives in the context of the external environment and an organization's internal strengths and weaknesses. When completed, it should include tactics, budgets, and timelines for achieving the strategic objectives.

So, how do you decide what technology you need for your organization?

The answer is two-fold. First, look at your strategic objectives and tactics. In what ways might technology help to achieve them? If so, how much will it cost? Secondly, when you or your staff trip across new software applications or the latest in application upgrades and cutting-edge technology, ask yourself this question: which, if any, of our strategic objectives would this technology help us achieve and is it worth the cost?

2. How Much Should We Be Spending on Technology?

In terms of budget allocations for information technology, health care has traditionally lagged behind other industries, with organizations spending only 2% to 4% of their budgets on information technology as compared to banking and finance industries which spend two to three times that amount. *The OPEN MINDS Report On Technology Applications In The Behavioral Health & Social Service Fields: The 2002 Survey Edition* indicates that, on average, the majority of organizations in our industry (23%) spent under $25,000 in the year 2000 on information technology, approximately an average of 4% of their budgets. Seventy-six percent of all organizations surveyed spent $300,000 or less on technology in 2000.

But are these benchmarks for technology spending useful in determining how much your organization should spend on technology?

The answer is both yes and no. Benchmark data is useful in giving you an overall sense of whether or not your

Behavioral Health & Social Service Organizations Technology Budgets, % By Organization Type - All Organizations Combined, 2000	
Up to $25,000	23%
$25,100 - $50,000	12%
$51,000 - $100,000	15%
$101,000 - $200,00	15%
$201,000 - $300,000	11%
$301,000 - $400,000	6%
$401,000 - $500,000	6%
$501,000 - $600,000	1%
$601,000 - $1 Million	5%
$1.1 Million - $3 Million	4%
$3.1 Million - $6 Million	1%
Over $6 Million	1%

organization is spending "enough" on IT, particularly if you use benchmarks for organizations of similar size and type. However, in markets where rapid change is occurring, organizations may need to spend significantly more on technology in order to be competitive or to meet the performance and reporting demands of the new marketplace, thus making the benchmark data less meaningful. Additionally, if your organization has historically under-budgeted technology, you may need to make considerable short-term investments in order to build the infrastructure necessary to do business in today's behavioral health and social service market.

So how much should your organization budget for technology? The right answer is fairly straightforward: whatever you need to achieve your organization's strategic objectives. When you have laid out an organizational strategy with clear objectives, you can determine what role technology can play in achieving them and can then proceed to budget for technology using a cost-benefit or return-on-investment model.

3. Should We Buy or Build the Technology We Need?

For most organizations, the answer to this technology question is easy. You should buy rather than build as long as you can purchase or piece together (via electronic data interfaces and/or data warehouses) the technology solution you need to get the functionality and benefits needed to run your organization and achieve your key strategic objectives. Decisions to build technology solutions — most commonly, software applications — are often driven by the following assumptions:

- Belief in organizational uniqueness — "We're so different from other organizations that no one has software that could meet our needs."
- Inability to restructure workflow to optimize the use of available technology —
  In this instance, an organization chooses to build technology to automate current processes rather than to make changes in process to use available technology.
- A lack of understanding the costs of building and maintaining an in-house technology solution — All costs must be included when budgeting for building technology solutions, including the costs of initial development

and testing, end-user and programmer documentation and training, report development, maintenance, and upgrades, etc.

For most organizations, building and maintaining technology is not a core competency nor is it central to their missions. Does this mean that it never makes sense to build rather than buy technology? No — if you can't buy or bundle available solutions, it may make sense to build the technology. Before doing so, however, it is important to rule out customization of available technologies (ideally through contracting with the vendor) or outsourcing as options and to ensure that your planning and budgeting for building the technology is complete.

Currently, there are two instances where behavioral health and social service organizations have been more likely to choose to build in-house software applications as technology solutions — if strategic business needs require managed care organization (MCO) functionality or if the organization is a child welfare provider. Presumably, this has been because there have historically been fewer technology vendors in the marketplace that offer products with the core functionality required in these cases.

Steps for Linking Organizational Strategy With Technology Planning

There is a six-step process for linking organizational strategy to your strategic technology planning:

Step 1: Develop a Strategic Business Plan with Clear Organizational Objectives and Tactics

Effective technology planning and budgeting can only occur if your organization has a well- formulated strategic plan with clear short-term and long-term strategic business objectives.

Step 2: Identify Opportunities Where Technology Is Needed to Achieve the Strategic Objectives

With a clear set of organizational objectives in place, the next step is to identify where technology can help out. This requires that you maintain a good understanding of available technologies in the industry as well as be able to envision how they might work for your organization. For example, is one of your objectives to streamline access to services so that you can improve satisfaction and increase revenues? If so, technology options may include enhanced phone system capabilities and software with scheduling functionality. See the chart on page 59 for other examples of how technology can help with common strategic objectives.

Step 3: Conduct Functionality Comparisons

The third step is to compare the functionality of the current technologies you have in place (if any) with those required for the proposed strategic objectives and tactics. Build a list of the functional enhancements that are needed.

Step 4: Estimate the Costs of Adding the Required Functionality in the Required Timeline

This is the research stage. Here you need to identify what options are currently available to put the required technology in place. Can you upgrade or customize current technology? Do you need to buy or build it? Is there an option to outsource to achieve the technological requirements? In instances where you are seeking major software applications, this stage may include a formal proposal and vendor selection process. The goals during this step are to select the technology solution(s) needed and to determine the total costs of getting them operational so the strategic objectives can be achieved in the required timeline.

Step 5: Incorporate Costs in the Budget Model to Test the Strategic Plan

This step is fairly uncomplicated. Simply load the cost information obtained in the previous step into your proposed budget.

Step 6: Proceed or Reject Technology Based Upon Budget Feasibility

Is the proposed organizational budget acceptable? If so, proceed with implementing the technologies selected. If not, the challenge is to rework the various budget and technology plan components in order to find an acceptable model. This might include modifying the technological functionality required or how it is purchased or obtained. Or, as in routine budget balancing acts, expense and revenue targets may need to be modified.

Aligning Technology with Your Organization's Strategic Objectives	
Strategic Objective	**Technology Options**
Improve access to care through centralized intake	Enhanced phone system capabilities
	Scheduling software
	Internet referral and service access options
Increase staff productivity	Electronic medical records
	Wireless input devices
	Automating repetitive tasks through practice management or MCO software applications
Increase profitability through unit cost management and target costing	Activity-based costing (ABC) software applications
Increase consumer use of self-help and natural support systems	On-line behavioral health databases
	Interactive Internet or computer-based self-help services
	Internet chat rooms and bulletin boards
Reduce hospitalization cost for consumers in rural areas by enhanced medication management	Video and telephone conferencing with psychiatrists and nurses
	E-mail

The New World of Technology Planning

As you can see, the proposed model for technology planning is quite different from how we've historically done things in behavioral health and social services. The old world approach was one where technology budgeting was somewhat anecdotal and based more on the desires of information systems staff and up-to-the-minute technologies rather than organizational strategy. Technology planning was done periodically, with objectives and timelines determined and driven only by the information systems staff. Oftentimes there was a discrepancy between what consumers or operational staff needed from technology and what was laid out in the plans developed by systems staff.

In the new world of technology planning, investments in technology are incorporated into the budgets set during the strategic planning process. The technology planning process is on-going with formal project management and key milestones and objectives. Additionally, the role of technology staff in the organization is different. They have on-going interaction with customers and operating teams, and they work in partnership with clinical and administrative staff in finding and successfully implementing the technologies needed to achieve organizational strategic and operational objectives.

What are the management implications and impacts of this new approach to technology planning? There are several:

- Organizations must keep abreast of the latest technologies available in order to maintain a competitive edge.
- Technology planning and budgeting must be incorporated into a formal strategic planning process, and implementation timelines will need to be aggressively managed in order to obtain the required functionality and achieve strategic objectives.
- On-going staff technology skill development and assessment will play an increasing role in human resource management.
- Data warehousing, outsourcing, partnering, or leasing technology will become increasingly attractive as options for obtaining needed technological capabilities. ▨

Return-On-Investment for Technology: A Decision Tool for Value-Based Purchasing for Behavioral Health & Social Service Executives

Joseph P. Naughton-Travers, Ed.M.

For most behavioral health and social service organizations, technology is a significant investment. Whether it's rolling out a major software application, putting computers and internet access on everyone's desktop, or implementing wireless technology to collect data from the field, the key question is often "Is this technology really worth the investment?"

Sometimes our technology investments are simply a part of doing business — such as beefing up our understaffed information technology departments and giving everyone computers, e-mail, and internet access. But, in other instances, we are looking for a way to guarantee the value and benefits we expect from the new technology. Will we really get improved clinical productivity if we implement that electronic medical records system? Will we be able to eliminate some clerical and billing staff by rolling out a superior practice management software application? Will wireless technology help us better manage our field staff and improve their productivity? Is this new technology really an investment or just a necessary business expense?

A common business approach — return-on-investment (ROI) analysis — can be used as a decision making tool to answer these types of questions and to ensure that your organization realizes the financial return that it expects in purchasing technology. Essentially, ROI is a formal process for quantifying the anticipated costs and benefits of the technology purchase, as well as the timeline within which they will occur. This article will cover the basics of a simple ROI approach to value-based technology purchasing, and how to use the tool and associated performance metrics to ensure that you achieve the intended results.

In general, return-on-investment analysis is likely to show significant financial return if the technology adopted has the following characteristics:

- Breadth: if there is widespread use of the technology throughout your organization (e.g., an integrated practice management, medical records, and general ledger software application that is used by all administrative and clinical staff)
- Complexity: if the technology automates complex work processes (e.g., editing service charges for payer billing rules and comparing services delivered to clinical best practice guidelines)
- Importance: if the work enhanced by the technology is critical to your organization (e.g., implementing a software application that aids in tracking real-time unit costs and quality measures)
- Collaboration: if the technology promotes communication and collaboration between departments and other stakeholders (e.g., wireless technology that allows clinicians working in the community to track critical risk factors and report services for billing)
- Reuse: if the technology helps to create an institutional memory where knowledge can be saved and reused (e.g., implementing a Help Desk software application that creates a database of problems and solutions over time)

The Basics of ROI for Technology Investments

Return-on-investment for technology is essentially a cost-benefit analysis. With it, you attempt to determine the benefits (focusing most heavily on the quantifiable ones that result in a financial return) as well as the costs involved in purchasing, implementing, and using the new technology. The formula for a simple ROI for a given time period is as follows:

- ROI = Net Benefit/Total Cost

For example, if you calculate $500,000 in financial benefits and $250,000 in costs for implementing the technology, this results in a 200% return-on-investment.

When doing an ROI analysis, there are a number of broad questions to consider:

What Will Be the Effect of the Technology Investment on Your Organization's Ability to Achieve Its Strategic and Operational Objectives?

Technology decision making should always be made in the context of your organization's overall planning process. We should be using technology as a tool to achieve organizational objectives, not for just for the sake of technology itself.

What Is the Cost of Implementation Over What Period in Time?

Typically, a return-on-investment analysis for a major technology initiative will cover a three year time period. The complete costs associated with purchasing and implementing the technology need be calculated.

Which of the Benefits of Technology Can Be Quantified and Which Cannot?

The financial and non-financial benefits of implementing the technology should be identified. The quantifiable ones will be used for the ROI analysis itself.

At What Point in the Implementation Will the Benefits Be Realized?

As with the costs, you will need to determine at what point in the implementation the financial benefits will be realized. Typically in a major technology implementation, you would expect to see some financial benefits after a six month period. In the event that you predict they will occur significantly later than this, it is recommended that you aggressively retool the implementation plan to ensure that you achieve some benefit during the first year of implementation.

What Performance Measures Can Be Monitored to Ensure That Actual Costs and Benefits Match Those Predicted in the ROI Analysis?

Lastly, as with all good financial planning processes, it is essential that you establish benchmarks and reporting capabilities to ensure that your organization achieves the calculated return-on- investment.

Calculating the Return-On-Investment for a Technology Purchase

So how do you perform a formal return-on-investment analysis for technology purchasing?

There are five basic steps:

- Step #1: Identify all costs associated with purchasing, implementing, and using the technology.
- Step #2: Identify quantifiable benefits associated with implementing the technology and the assumptions these benefits are based on.
- Step #3: Determine the timing (usually by month or quarter) of each of the categories of cost and financial benefit.
- Step #4: Calculate the overall return-on-investment, as well as the costs and benefits for each financial time period, and modify the plan as needed.
- Step #5: Develop and implement performance measures, benchmarks, and/or reporting systems to ensure the ROI is achieved.

Technology ROI Analysis Assumptions

- Definition: The financial return (or benefit) derived from an investment in technology
- The technology investment is being made to improve financial performance and/or reduce costs
- Simple ROI formula: ROI = net benefit/total cost

Step #1: Identify All Costs Associated With Purchasing, Implementing, and Using the Technology

This is usually the easiest step. The key to Step #1 is to determine all one-time and on-going costs associated with implementing the new technology. These costs usually fall into the following categories:

- Hardware: These include computers, printers, file servers, wireless devices, and other required equipment.

- Hardware Maintenance: These include any additional costs associated with repair and service of the required hardware.
- Connectivity: These include any one-time and on-going costs such as internet connections, telecommunication and frame-relay services, wireless connectivity, etc.
- Software Licenses or User Fees: These include either one-time license fees or the monthly user fees typically associated with application service provider (ASP) vendors. Additionally, be certain to include fees for the purchase of any required third-party software products (such as Microsoft Windows, Crystal Reports, etc.) needed to use the chosen technology.
- Installation & Customization: Typically, these are one-time fees for customizing and installing the technology.
- Data Migration: These are fees associated with extracting data from one software application and migrating it into the new technology. This is typically done to save time when implementing practice management or managed care organization software applications.
- Staff Training: This should include both the initial and on-going training for staff in using the technology.
- Software Maintenance & Upgrades: Ideally, these are annual fees for receiving all software enhancements, bug fixes, and upgrades. In some instances, upgrades are charged separately from routine enhancements and bug fixes.
- User Support: This should include the cost of vendor support (usually on an hourly basis or as part of a monthly support fee) in addition to the costs for any internal Help Desk (typically staff and software) that your organization implements.
- Additional Information Technology Staff: This would include any additional staff your organization needs to maintain and support the new technology.

Step #2: Identify Quantifiable Benefits Associated with Implementing the Technology and the Assumptions These Benefits Are Based On

Identifying the financial benefits of implementing the technology — though fairly straightforward — is a bit trickier. The key here is to ensure that the financial returns are both realistic and realizable. Typically, the benefits from implementing the use of technology in the behavioral health and social service industry fall into four broad categories:

- Reduced Labor Costs Through Automation: This is the most common category of financial benefit for implementing technology — reducing the number of staff members through automation. This may include staff who perform functions including medical records transcription, data entry, and manual data gathering and report generation.
- Additional Revenues Through Increased Productivity: This would include any additional revenues generated through improved productivity for clinical staff members.
- Reduced Compliance & Accreditation Costs: These occur most commonly when implementing an electronic medical record (EMR). They typically include expectation of reduced recoupments from payers for better compliance with medical record requirements and the reduced cost of preparing for accreditation reviews.
- Improved Collections & Payment Turnaround Time: These benefits occur when implementing technologies with enhanced third-party billing capabilities. Accounts receivable collection and payment turnaround time is usually improved by better edits for compliance with payer billing regulations, electronic billing, and improved management reporting.

How do you best estimate the financial benefits of implementing the technology in these four areas? Most technology vendors will tell you about expected savings and benefits, but the key is to determine whether or not your organization will really achieve them.

- Can you contact other customers who have implemented the chosen technology?
  If so, what financial benefits did they achieve? Which did they expect, yet not realize?
- If you predict savings through automation, will your organization really eliminate full or partial staff positions?
- If you are expecting increased revenues through productivity enhancement, how will you ensure that they occur?
- Do you have enough information about current compliance costs and collection efforts to make accurate assumptions about improvements in these areas?

Step #3: Determine the Timing (Usually by Month or Quarter) of Each of the Categories of Cost and Financial Benefit

Once you've finalized your list of expected financial benefits, you can move to Step #3 — determining the timing of the various costs and the benefits of the technology. Typically this is done in a spreadsheet, much like any budgeting process.

Step #4: Calculate the Overall Return-On-Investment, as well as the Costs and Benefits for Each Financial Time Period, and Modify the Plan as Needed

This allows you to make the calculations needed in Step #4 — the overall return-on-investment, as well as the costs and benefits (and hence the cash flow requirements), for each fiscal period. At this point, you may also need to rework the ROI budget to meet your financial requirements.

Step #5: Develop and Implement Performance Measures, Benchmarks, and/or Reporting Systems to Ensure the ROI Is Achieved

The last step for the analysis is to build a management process to ensure that the expected return-on-investment is achieved. This typically includes performance reporting (e.g., productivity and collection percentages), benchmarks and milestones (e.g., when certain positions are expected to be eliminated as automation occurs), and management reporting to compare ROI actual and budgeted costs and benefits.

Tips for Putting Together an Effective Return-On-Investment Analysis

Return-on-investment analysis is an effective business tool not only because it helps to answer the question "should we buy this technology?" but also because the process requires an organization to focus on its functional needs and expected benefits from using the technology, as well as the timeline within which they should be achieved. When you embark on an ROI analysis for technology, keep the following tips in mind:

- Start with a strategic focus on technology — how it will help your organization achieve desired strategic and operational objectives.

- Bring information technology, finance, and clinical operations staff together to develop the ROI assumptions and model.
- Be conservative in your assumptions of financial benefits.
- Build a technology implementation timeline that accelerates the time period when the benefits kick in.
- Set clear milestones and performance metrics to ensure that the expected return and benefits are achieved. ▨

Strategic Management

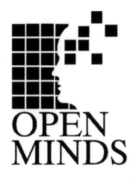

OPEN
MINDS

Data-Driven Decision-Making: Moving to an Organizational Measurement Culture

Joseph P. Naughton-Travers, Ed.M.

Success in business planning and management requires that we move from a traditional model of providing purely financial and retrospective information and using best guesses for decision making to one of providing forward looking and insightful measurement and analysis that can be used to make key decisions. I call this a measurement culture — where business decisions are made based upon a careful blend of both data and intuition. It is an organizational environment where staff have a keen understanding of the information they need to do their jobs effectively and how to obtain and use this data. It is a culture where organizational performance is driven by measuring, reporting, and managing key strategic and operational metrics.

How do we transform our organizations into this sort of measurement culture?

Essentially, there are three key components necessary to accomplish this:
- An information infrastructure where staff have access to accurate, up-to-date data for making management decisions
- A formal performance measurement system where selected strategic and operational metrics are reported on a monthly basis
- Standard reporting of selected performance metrics and compliance data to executive management and the board of directors so they can fulfill their roles in providing organizational oversight and strategic direction

This article details these three required components for developing an organizational measurement culture, as well as the related human resource challenges.

Building a Foundation for Data-Driven Decision-Making

Before you can transform your organization to one that focuses on measurement and data for making management decisions, you must first build the infrastructure necessary to gather and disseminate information. The goal here is to make certain that all staff have access to the accurate, up-to-date information that they need to do their jobs on a daily basis. For most organizations, this means producing and using meaningful reports from the management information system.

Why do so many organizations struggle with this?

Most often, the reason is that many behavioral health and social service organizations still primarily use their management information system for billing and financial functions, not as a true information system. You can begin to change this by first focusing on the desired end results — the information that staff need to do their jobs. What data do they need and when do they need it? Are you even collecting this data in your MIS? What report layouts are needed to communicate the desired information? Does your MIS generate these reports, or do they need to be developed?

As a starting point for identifying your reporting needs, see the chart on page 79 for a listing of routine reports used by behavioral health and social service providers and managed care organizations.

Once you have identified the routine management reports your staff need, the next steps for building this foundation for data-driven decision making and management are as follows:

- Ensure you are collecting all of the data needed to generate routine management reports.
- Institute data accuracy checks to ensure the integrity of the information.
- Develop new reports as needed and establish a schedule for report generation to ensure staff receive their reports when they need them.
- Train staff to read and use the reports.

Implementing a Formal Performance Measurement System

Having an effective and efficient information infrastructure in place is not enough to transform your organization into a true measurement culture. The next step is to institute a formal performance measurement reporting system, with financial and non-financial metrics that can be used by managers in ensuring that the organization is moving forward in achieving its strategic and operational objectives. Most commonly known as key performance indicators (KPIs), these metrics are used by executive leadership to communicate strategy and focus, and they become vital in making proactive management decisions.

A "balanced scorecard" is a best-practice approach to performance measurement. With it, your organization focuses on measurements which reflect four key business perspectives:

- Financial: These measures reflect the overall financial status of your organization.
- Customer: These measures reflect customer satisfaction (consumer, payer, network provider, and other stakeholders) with your organization's services.
- Innovation: These measures reflect your organization's commitment to acquiring and implementing new knowledge.
- Internal Operations: These measures reflect the overall health of your organization's internal departments and processes.

See the chart below and on the next two pages for examples of performance measures in these four categories.

Routine Management Information Reports for Behavioral Health & Social Service Organizations		
	Report	Description
Finance	Aged Trial Balance	Details the accounts receivable
	Pre-Billing Edit	Warns staff about services that have not cleared the information system's edits regarding payer rules
	General Ledger Posting	Details the G/L account entries necessary for posting month end financial data into the accounting system
	Deposit Reconciliation	Details deposits and checks posted in the information system
	Collection	Provides detailed service and consumer information for unpaid claims so that collection and follow-up activity can occur
	Bad Debt Write-Offs	Details the dollar amounts and reasons for bad debt write-offs
	Day in A/R	Calculates the average number of days from billing to payment for selected claim types
	Collection Percentage	Calculates the percentage of the net accounts receivable collected thus far for selected claim types

Routine Management Information Reports for Behavioral Health & Social Service Organizations	
Report	**Description**

	Report	Description
Clinical	Diagnostic Profile	Summarizes diagnostic mix for select consumers
	Service Mix Profile	Summarizes service mix for select consumers
	Length of Treatment	Summarizes length of treatment (visits or days) for select consumers
	Psychotropic Medication Profile	Summarizes psychotropic medications used by select consumers
Operations	Active Consumer List	Details consumers currently in care
	Consumer Service History	Details service history for a single consumer
	Care Referrals	Details referral sources, reasons, and dispositions
	Missing Consumer Data	Alerts staff to missing consumer data elements required for operations
	Missing Service Authorizations	Alerts staff of services scheduled or rendered which are missing required service authorizations
	Service Authorization Warning	Alerts staff of service authorizations that will be depleted in the near future
	Caseload by Care Provider	Summarizes caseload for each care provider
	Productivity Management	Compares clinical staff productivity against productivity standards
	Cancellations & No-Shows	Details consumer cancellations and no-shows by site and care provider
	Medical Record Tickler	Alerts staff of required medical records tasks
	Appointment Schedule	Details ambulatory appointment schedule
	Satisfaction & Outcomes	Details consumer satisfaction and outcomes by site and care provider
	Credentialing Tickler Warning	Reminds staff of the need to re-credential care providers
Care Management Programs	Hospital Admission	Details consumers authorized and admitted for hospital level care
	Care Access Decisions	Details access center referrals and dispositions
	Service Denial/Reduction	Details service authorization request denials or reductions
	Provider Authorization Appeals	Details appeals regarding authorization decisions
	Capitation Financial Management	Details revenues and expenses for a capitated contract
	Claims Processing	Summarizes claims adjudication processing, including paid, pending, and denied claims
	IBNR	Calculates "incurred but not reported" claims to estimate financial liability for network provider services
	Network Provider Performance	Details performance measures for network providers
	Satisfaction & Outcomes	Details consumer satisfaction and outcomes for select network providers
	Credentialing & Privileging Tickler	Reminds staff of the need to re-credential or re-privilege network providers
	Member Complaints	Details consumer complaints
	Grievance & Appeals Status	Details grievances and appeals
	Penetration	Details service penetration for member population

The main point is that focusing on financial metrics is not enough. The key to long-term organizational success is to select a combination of both financial and non-financial metrics that both drive performance improvement and identify problem areas for management intervention. Key performance indicator measures are reported for the current month as well as the previous 12 months to aid in identifying trends and instituting corrective actions or special studies.

Commonly Used Performance Measurement Metrics	
Measurement Category	**Sample Metrics**
Financial	Profit & Loss by Service Line Budget Variance by Service Line Cost Per Unit of Service
Customer	Number of Consumers Served by Service Line Number of Consumer Complaints Successful Discharges by Program Percentage of Consumers with Improved Functioning Average Consumer Satisfaction Average Employee Satisfaction Market Share by Service Line Number of Authorization Appeals (MCO) Number of Grievances (MCO) Grievance & Appeals Overturn Rates (MCO) Number of Network Provider Complaints (MCO)
Innovation	Number of Staff Training Days Number of Community Educations Hours Percentage of Revenues from New Service Lines Number of Positive Media Mentions
Internal Operations	Average Number of Days to Care Access by Service Line Data Entry Procedural Accuracy Rolling Staff Turnover Rate (3-month) Percentage of Claims Denied Collection Percentages for Third-Party Billings Bad Debt Write-Offs Percentage of Employees Who Met Productivity Standards Claims Inventory (MCO)

As you begin to implement a performance measurement system, keep the following in mind:

- Make certain that you select metrics that measure progress towards key strategic objectives for your organization as well as operational metrics for departments where you know there is need for improvement.
- Set targets or standards for the performance metrics.

- Seek out industry benchmarks for selected metrics so that you can drive performance improvement.
- Modify the KPI metrics as needed, and consider publishing a "community report card" periodically with selected metrics.

What's Different About the Data Needed by Boards of Directors

Your board of directors should also receive some version of a key performance indicator report. It is succinct and — if the metrics are well-selected — should summarize the overall health of the organization and its progress towards strategic objectives. However, because of its governing role in an organization, the board of directors needs more than just performance data. It also needs compliance and risk management data to ensure that your organization has met its legal and contractual obligations. This compliance reporting, in conjunction with the strategic performance measures are the critical information needed by the board for decision making.

This compliance and risk management reporting reflect the responsibility for the following:
- Growing number of federal and state regulations with regard to operations, performance, and reporting
- Increasing and changing state and local reporting requirements
- Evolving accreditation and licensure requirements
- Contract-specific performance and reporting requirements

The key purpose of this type of reporting is to prevent fines, legal actions, or loss of contracts due to non-compliance with legal or contractual obligations. Boards of directors usually mandate that organizations develop formal corporate compliance programs in line with the requirements set out by the Office of Inspector General at the U.S. Department of Health and Human Services.

The suggested components for this compliance reporting to the board of directors include the following:

- Periodic data summarizing audits in the four key areas of greatest compliance risk for behavioral health provider and managed care organizations:
  - Billing and claims payment
  - Medical record documentation
  - Admissions and referral mechanisms
  - Provider credentialing and contracting
- Summaries of reported compliance violations and subsequent actions
- An annual report that informs the board of the strengths and weaknesses of the compliance program and how it should be altered to prevent violations in the future

Developing Information Literacy

This article has covered the three key components needed to move your organization to a measurement culture where management decisions are based on data, not just instinct. With routine management reports in place, along with a performance measurement and compliance reporting system, your staff, management and executive team, and board of directors should have access to the information they need to do their jobs effectively.

But there is a human resource issue at hand here too. We can't just focus on the tools and infrastructure necessary to support a measurement culture. We must actively invest acquiring or developing "information literacy" in our staff. Being information literate is not about becoming a technical computer guru (yet all staff must be comfortable with computer basics to survive in today's workplace). It is a skill set that involves understanding how to find and use information to do one's job. An information literate person knows what information he or she needs, how to get it, and how to use it most effectively to meet management needs and your organization's objectives. Only when you invest in the human side of the data and performance systems will you be able to successfully become an organization with a measurement culture. ▣

Strategic Management Competency

Using Information Systems to Develop Clinical Performance Scorecards: Reporting Behavioral Health & Social Service Clinical Team Performance

Robert M. Atkins, M.D., M.P.H.

Behavioral health organizations purchase information systems for a variety of reasons. These include streamlining financial processes, client billing and scheduling, and improving operating efficiencies. Information systems often have modular structures that address each of these functions and integrate data to enable sole source data entry that supports all downstream functions. Perhaps the most elusive goal, however, is using data entered into the system to improve your organization's clinical performance and productivity. A number of systemic barriers present in most organizations decrease the likelihood of this occurring. This article will identify the most common of these barriers and offer some recommendations for removing or minimizing these barriers to get the most from your current information system investment.

Erroneous Assumption: Performance Metrics Is a Compliance Requirement

The widespread assumption that reporting performance metrics is primarily a compliance requirement is the first barrier to successful use of your information system for metrics-based clinical performance improvement. Financial accounting statements, utilization measures, operational performance measures, continuous quality performance indicator (CQI) satisfaction surveys, and other outcome indicators are all reports that are often required by one or more stakeholders. For this reason, performance measurement is often compartmentalized in finance and quality assurance departments. This assumption suggests that leadership's role is to assure these compliance requirements are met, and then to move on to the real business of managing the organization.

There are two root causes impeding adoption of performance metrics as a management tool. The first is widespread discomfort with using quantitative data to drive clinical decision making and promote accountability. "Innumeracy" is analogous to illiteracy. It is a term coined by Douglas R. Hofstadter, director of the Center for Research on Concepts and Cognition at Indiana University and popularized by mathematician John Allen Paulos in a best-selling book of the same name. Innumeracy suggests an inability to think quantitatively, to interpret quantitative information in order to analyze and solve problems. This inability or unwillingness to apply mathematical ideas involving numbers or logic makes it impossible to use quantitative reasoning or to recognize meaningful quantitative patterns. The large number of behavioral health organizations that do not use their data to drive decisions suggests widespread management innumeracy.

The second root cause is that information systems may not meet the needs of clinical users. When designing, configuring, and implementing a new information system, administrators (and IT vendors) often begin with finance and business office operations. These departments are relatively easy to computerize, and these users typically are comfortable with computers. Then administration tries to get clinicians to use systems designed around financial and business office functions. When information systems do not collect data that is critical for clinical decision making, and do not support clinical workflow, clinicians are less likely to value those systems. Clinicians end up serving the system by entering data, but such systems may not serve the clinicians by returning useful reports.

The Business Perspective Versus the Clinical Perspective

The second barrier to data-driven performance is the great divide between clinical and administrative leadership. Administrative leadership is often focused on financial viability, while clinical leadership is focused on quality of care.

Both perspectives identify boundary conditions ("out-of-bounds") and an ultimate goal, and both use performance metrics as a way to assess movement toward the goal. But, they differ in their priorities. Both perspectives recognize the need to meet all compliance requirements: legal, regulatory, contractual, and ethical. They differ in that the business perspective requires "good enough" quality of care while maximizing financial viability, as measured by such parameters as operating margin and revenue growth. The clinical perspective requires "good enough" financial viability while maximizing quality of care, as measured by such parameters as community tenure and enhanced recovery. Executive leadership is more inclined to adopt the business perspective, because their concern is ultimately with staying in business and they understand financial data more than they understand clinical data. In addition, clinical leadership may rely more on anecdote and opinion rather than clinical performance data to drive decisions, which is less persuasive to executive leadership. The critical change in thinking is to show how to balance these two perspectives using performance measurement.

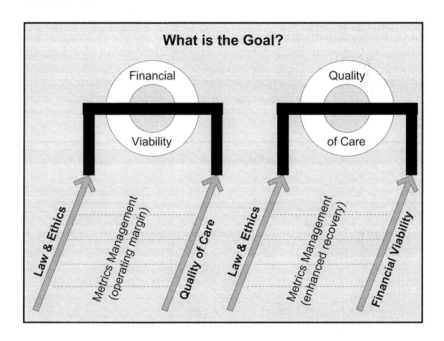

Can You Believe It?

With this divide, can you use your current information system to develop clinical performance scorecards — and drive clinical program and productivity improvement? The answer is "yes." The challenge is to identify what data is available and useful as proven indicators of clinical performance. The key is to create a scorecard clinicians will find useful. When people doubt the validity of a measurement, they will not use it constructively but simply see it as a requirement. If it is okay, they ignore it; if not, they create a corrective action plan to make it okay. Simply put, if a measurement isn't credible, people will produce it (compliance) but not use it to manage.

For purposes of measuring performance, metrics management is a system of related measures that quantifies the most important characteristics of your organization. With this in mind, there are four common examples of invalid ways to design a metric that will not be credible and could do harm by driving decisions that misallocate resources and fail to produce results. They are: drawing conclusions solely from numerator data; using an inappropriate denominator; comparing two measurements at two points in time; and using averages as the only metric to report performance

Drawing conclusions from only numerator data is usually meaningless for comparing performance or for tracking and trending performance over time. Except in the case of a sentinel event, where every instance is cause for concern, simple counts have little value in driving improvement. Knowing the number of complaints, or the number of errors, or the number of abandoned calls, is simply raw data that has not yet been transformed into useful information. For most indicators the raw count requires some way to normalize the data that accounts for important differences between comparison groups and over time. This requires selecting a denominator.

Using an inappropriate denominator will misrepresent the data and can lead to bad management decisions. A denominator should represent the true area of opportunity for the numerator event to occur. Selecting a denominator that appears logical but does not represent the true area of opportunity is a common error that produces a distorted picture of actual performance. For example, the number of medical necessity denials per month is a common metric, but assumes that the number of units of service that could potentially be denied remains essentially the same month to month. While this may be reasonable for an inpatient unit that hovers at close to 100% throughout the year, it is less likely to portray actual performance in an outpatient clinic. It may be more useful to report the number of actual units of service denied divided by the number of units of service delivered. This definition of a denial rate takes into account changes in volume over time, which would confound the denials per month metric.

Comparing two measurements at two points in time ignores the natural variation present in any process over time. While any two numbers are almost certain to be different, the real question is whether the difference is meaningful. When tracking and trending system performance over time, it is critical to compare two periods of sustained performance to identify a shift in baseline. Point-to-point comparisons reveal little about the effectiveness of the management intervention.

Using averages as the only metric to report performance is nearly ubiquitous, and contains four common errors: reporting average performance without any measure of dispersion; blending performance of different populations into an overall average; combining incommensurate units into a single number; and including outliers in reporting average system performance.

Reporting average performance without any measure of dispersion, such as the range or standard deviation, ignores the natural variation that is inherent to every process. "Metrics management" means using metrics as a management tool to assure performance meets requirements and to improve performance. This is impossible without knowing the range within which actual performance varies and comparing this to the target or threshold that desired performance must meet.

Blending performance of different populations into an overall average is not statistically valid. Using metrics in real-world situations, unlike research settings, means the subjects being measured are heterogeneous in all kinds of ways. A group of people, say everyone receiving inpatient treatment over a twelve-month period, is almost certainly comprised of subpopulations that are meaningful to the metric being reported. For example, acute inpatient units might include Medicare recipients with an average length of stay (ALOS) of 30 days, and non-Medicare recipients with an ALOS of six days. Changes in the unit's ALOS might be caused by changes in the relative mix of these two subpopulations and no change in clinical performance. To report a blended ALOS and assume changes are due to clinical performance is unlikely to be credible to clinicians on the unit.

Combining incommensurate units into a single number is another frequently occurring error. Behavioral health treatment includes many different types of units of service, such as medication injections, medication management visits, psychotherapy sessions, and inpatient days. To calculate an average unit cost by adding the total number of units of service of all types and then dividing by the total costs has no meaning. While mathematically sound, this number is useless to management. But this method of measurement is surprisingly common.

Including outliers in reporting average system performance skews the data and compromises its value in understanding how to improve performance. In clinical practice, we know that there are a small number of people with unusual circumstances, or with treatment resistant or complex disorders, who are exceptional. Measured performance related to these individuals is less a function of how the system works and more a function of what it is that makes each one exceptional. Routine measures of system performance should identify and exclude such exceptional individuals, commonly described as outliers.

Recommendations

In order to use your current information system to develop clinical performance scorecards, it is critical to adopt a systems thinking perspective to understand your organization. Viewing your organization as a system means understanding how each key function serves the needs of its internal and external customers. This lays the foundation for recognizing that clinicians are the ultimate internal customers of many of your system's processes and that the systemic constraint on your organization's productivity is the capacity of your clinical staff to deliver high value treatment and services. This makes it critical to subordinate all other operational processes to maximize clinician efficiency, thereby getting the most out of the constraining component of your system, and making the best use of current resources. (This insight comes from the work of Eliyahu M. Goldratt and his Theory of Constraints.) If clinicians are the ultimate internal customers of the information system, then their requirements should be the first consideration, not the last. The information system must comply with the requirements for finance and business office operations, but the goal is to maximize clinical performance.

The next recommendation is for every manager to become a skilled metrics manager and learn to generate, analyze, interpret, and make routine use of financial, operational, and clinical performance metrics. This should be an explicit management core competency for everyone in a management role, including all clinical managers. It requires understanding process variation and using CQI methods such as pareto analysis and statistical process control as a way of thinking and as analytical tools.

Finally, get your staff involved in all aspects of performance measurement by giving an overview briefing and regular updates, showing the benefit to the organization and ultimately to them. Explain how they can help by collecting good data. Make them aware of the potential for bad management decisions that could adversely impact them if data is not accurate. Make it personal by tying performance goals directly to their personal performance and identify clear rewards, i.e., bonuses, promotions, or other perks for peak performance. Management decisions that influence the future of the organization and consequently affect every staff member must be based on sound data. Assuring the accuracy and usefulness of the data should be the goal of every staff member.

In summary, I have discussed the three most common barriers to getting optimal use of your information system to measure and improve clinical performance; four errors in designing metrics, which can render them useless; and four common mistakes to avoid when using averages. Recognizing these barriers is the first step towards overcoming them. Train your managers to be conversant with statistics, involve your staff, and collect good data, and you will be successful in using your information system to develop viable clinical performance scorecards. ▨

Strategic Management Competency

Not-For-Profit Execs Face Issue of Greatest Good With Limited Resources: Balancing Social Mission, Community Expectations & Available Funding

Monica E. Oss, M.S.

"The challenge for non-profit human service leadership today is to turn mission-driven organizations into businesses with a mission." Those are the words of an executive with a not-for-profit children's agency, and they summarize succinctly the challenge that lies ahead for many not-for-profit behavioral health and social service organizations. Unfortunately, the reality is far more difficult than the platitude. Certainly, good management practices make precious charitable resources go further, and there are many management practices common in the for-profit community of which not-for-profit executives could make good use. But there is a level of complexity in relationship with payers, in organizational change, and with community expectations that make this a very difficult task. Providing not-for-profit (NFP) directors, executives, and staff with quantitative information on organizational performance that can be used in decision-making is a first step in an evolutionary process to enhance NFP strategy development for the years ahead.

Most CEOs of not-for-profit organizations in the field don't relish the prospect of remaking their management infrastructure. But, the past dozen years have changed the strategic environment in our field. Not-for-profit organizations in behavioral health and social services are increasingly dependent upon government, as opposed to charitable, funding — funds which are increasingly awarded using competitive procurement and risk-based or performance-based contracting practices. There is also more competition for charitable contributions, coupled with increasing donor skepticism of not-for-profit organizations. (While Enron was making the headlines at press time, the non-profit world has its own Hale House scandal brewing.) In addition, accessing foundation resources and grant funding has become increasing complicated.

At the same time, a combination of public policy decisions and a weakening economy have created more demand for government-funded services at a time when this funding is decreasing. The historical environment was characterized by cost-plus reimbursement and program funding with little accountability, with charitable contributions providing the "extras" as opposed to the "essentials". The current environment is very different. Organizations face an environment with lower fees, unfunded public policy mandates, and increasing administrative burden related to both compliance and accountability. Charitable contributions have moved from "extras" to "essentials". Cost-shifting from both private and public payers to financially unsophisticated not-for-profit organizations is now typical.

The question for many NFP boards of directors and management teams is at what point the burden of cost-shifting is greater than the resources of an individual agency to continue to serve the community. These executives need to decide whether charitable dollars should subsidize public and/or private payers. And if so, what are the limits to the charitable dollars available to supplement the shortfall between public policy and public spending? In my work with NFP boards and management teams in our field, I think they now have the weighty obligation of answering the following four strategic questions:

1. Is my organization a 'good steward' of public and charitable funds?
2. Does my organization provide 'better value' for these funds than other service organizations?
3. To best fulfill our mission in the community, what services should my organization provide?
4. Of those services, which consumers and/or consumer services should be subsidized with charitable dollars if government funding only covers a portion of the costs — and to what degree?

Managing Non-Profit Organizations Is Different ... A Question of Complex Financing & Complex Expectations

Management tools 'borrowed' from for-profit organizations can certainly enhance the ability of NFP executives to make informed choices. At a minimum, I think all behavioral health and social service organizations need resource-based strategic planning tools, unit cost management initiatives, key performance measurement reporting at all organizational levels, return-on-investment methodologies for making investments in systems and facilities, and a rule-based subsidy allocation system. However, improving the management infrastructure is a far simpler task than developing sustainable organizational policies and procedures to address the issue of finite charitable contributions and almost limitless community need. There are two factors that make rational management and decision-making processes difficult — the complexity of non-profit financing in behavioral health and social services and the conflicts between the organization's mission, community expectations of the organization, and available funding.

Most organizations in the health and human service field exist in an environment of mandated complexity. In many states, the payment to provider organizations for the delivery of consumer services is an odd mix of deficit-funded program fees, Medicaid reimbursement rates, specific grant funding, county contributions, and payments from care management organizations. More often than not, the financing modes conflict (with no flexibility to provide the 'right service' for consumers or to find economies of scale) — and the reporting requirements are duplicative and often nonsensical. The various programs, initiatives, and regulations that have lead to these types of situations were often very well-intended. But, the political rigor mortise that has caused this complexity does not result in better consumer service, nor does it provide an environment where standard management tools can have their greatest positive effect.

The long-term net effect of the intersection of politics and conflicting public policy has left the front-line providers of consumer service in an unenviable position: high administrative costs because of duplicative and conflicting reporting and billing requirements, financial reporting requirements that do not support cost management initiatives, and unclear performance expectations. Like it or not, many management teams are stuck with that complex environment — the question is how to apply best practices in organizational management to this environment.

Another difficult issue for NFP executives is managing conflicting sets of expectations. The for-profit world and the government world are far simpler. Making a profit, innovative programming with high market-share and high levels of customer satisfaction and loyalty are consistent performance objectives in the for-profit world. Balancing budgets, meeting mandated requirements and political success are consistent themes in the government sector. But, for NFP executives and boards, the signals are a bit mixed. Organizational missions, community expectations, the requirements of government funding agencies, and the goals of charitable donors are rarely in sync. In fact, they are often in direct conflict. A key role for NFP board leadership today is aligning the organization's mission and the expectations of the community with the realities of available funding from both government and charitable sources. With that difficult alignment, and not to be underestimated, is the task of preparing for a change in organizational culture as long-time consumers, staff, community stakeholders, and directors themselves adjust to all that these changes imply.

Developing an Organizational Measurement Culture as a Tool to Assure Good Stewardship and to Support Tough Choices

After a decade of working with NFPs in our field, both as a consultant and as a board member, I think that the changes in public policy and the environment have increased the need for NFP to move to an organizational "measurement culture". Quantitative information (about consumers, payers, financial performance, costs, operational systems, outcomes, and more) is key to facilitating good decision-making at the executive level. Answering the four strategic questions above is almost impossible without a basic set of metrics.

(Some recommended organizational performance metrics for board members are shown in the table on following page.)

Organizational Metrics Supporting Strategic Decision-Making in NFP Health & Human Service Environment	
Monthly NFP Organizational Performance Metric	**Description**
Income/Revenue, By Source & Service Line	Itemization of the income/revenue received from every payer source in total and by organizational service line.
Direct Expenses, By Service Line	Itemization of direct expenses for the organization in total and as assigned to an individual service line.
Allocated Expenses, By Service Line	Itemization of expenses other than direct expenses, along with assignment/allocation by service line.
Allocated Charitable Income/Revenue, By Service Line	Allocation of charitable incomes/revenue, by service line.
Profit/Loss By Services Line Without Charitable Allocation	Profit/loss of organization and of each service line without charitable resource allocation.
Total Profit/Loss By Service Line	Profit/loss of organization and of each service line.
Total # Of Clients Served, By Service Line & Relevant Demographic/Payer Type	Number of clients served in period, in total and by service line. Data reported by specific types of consumer demographics and/or payer type, as needed.
Total # Of Service Units Delivered, By Service Unit Type, By Service Line & By Relevant Demographic/Payer Type	Number of service units delivered by type. Data reported by service line and by specific types of consumer demographics and/or payer type, as needed.
Staff/Facility Productivity Or Yield, By Service Unit and/or Appropriate Operation Units	Staff/facility productivity or yield, by service unit and/or operational cost. Definitions of productivity or yield (available hours, available beds, billable hours, etc.) dependent on services and organization. Productivity or yield can be reported at whatever level is most useful for management — individual staff member, work teams, operational units, geographic locations, etc.
Total Direct Cost Per Service Unit, By Service Unit Type	Total direct costs for delivery of a particular type of service, by unit delivered.
Total Indirect Cost Per Service Unit	Total indirect costs for delivery of a particular type of service, by unit delivered

Organizational Metrics Supporting Strategic Decision-Making in NFP Health & Human Service Environment	
Monthly NFP Organizational Performance Metric	**Description**
Total Cost Per Service Unit	Total direct and indirect costs for delivery of a particular type of service, by unit delivered.
Non-Charitable Incomes/Revenue Per Service Unit	Non-charitable revenue/income received for delivery of a particular type of service, by unit delivered.
Charitable Income/Revenue Per Service Unit (Per Unit Subsidy)	Charitable revenue/income received for delivery of a particular type of service, by unit delivered.
Total Income/Revenue Per Service Unit	Total revenue/income received for delivery of a particular type of service, by unit delivered.
Profit/Loss Per Service Unit	Comparison of total revenue per service unit delivered to total cost per service unit delivered.
Subsidy As % of Total Cost Per Service Unit	Charitable income/revenue per service unit as a % of total cost.
Consumer Satisfaction/Outcome Measures, By Service Line	Consumer satisfaction and outcome measures, by service line. Most often established using existing satisfaction and outcome tools, with reporting by service line, service unit, and appropriate consumer demographic or organization characteristics.

In the current environment, the NFP directors and executives are the "front line" of rationing decisions. Access to these metrics allows executives and directors to develop strategies that focus organizations where they are most effective, to improve or discontinue ineffective programs or programs where the organization is no longer the 'best value' provider in the community, and to address issues of economies of scale. The economy of scale issue is a most pressing one. Many organizations are too small (in terms of both capital for investment and on-going administrative overhead) to maintain their current programs, and structure in the years ahead. It is likely that these organizations, even if they grow, will need to shed some programs and funding streams to focus resources and gain necessary economies of scale. For some, growth by merger and/or acquisition may be the best strategic choice. This is not possible to gauge without critical organizational and environmental data.

To further both mission and good stewardship, management teams in the current NFP health and human service environment should focus on putting the organization's financial and operational "house in order" by borrowing best practice quantitative tools for understanding both internal operations and the external environment. Use of these tools is the first step to moving to an organizational measurement culture that supports mission-based entrepreneurship in health and human services. ◪

Contributing Authors' Biographies

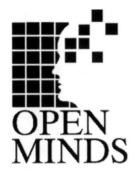

OPEN
MINDS

Robert M. Atkins, M.D., M.P.H

Robert M. Atkins, M.D., M.P.H, Advisory Board Member, has over twenty years experience in the management of behavioral health programs in the private and public sector. Dr. Atkins brings a wealth of experience to *OPEN MINDS* clients including executive experience in managed care, clinical risk management, and public mental health quality improvement.

Dr. Atkins is currently the chief medical officer at Advantage Care Select in Indianapolis. He was a medical director for Schaller Anderson, providing mental health policy consultation to state governments. He formerly served as regional medical director of the Louisville Region of Magellan Behavioral Health, where he designed and implemented a comprehensive regional prevention program in conformity with NCQA standards. Dr. Atkins was the chief executive officer and medical director of ClearSprings Health Partnership, where he reversed a 39% operating loss to a 12% net gain in a 12-month period. In addition, he has directed and assisted in the reengineering of numerous existing programs, resulting in increased quality of service and efficiencies, both financial and operational. Earlier in his career he was on the staff of a state psychiatric facility.

Dr. Atkins has held numerous academic appointments, serving as an assistant clinical professor of psychiatry and behavioral sciences at the University of Louisville School of Medicine; as clinical assistant professor and clinical instructor at the University of Maryland Hospital; and as an instructor at Johns Hopkins University. He received his Bachelor's degree from Franklin and Marshall College in Lancaster, Pennsylvania, his Doctor of Medicine (M.D.) from Johns Hopkins School of Medicine and his Master of Public Health (M.P.H.) from the Johns Hopkins School of Hygiene and Public Health. He is a board certified psychiatrist and is currently licensed to practice medicine in Kentucky and Tennessee. 🔳

Contributing Author

M. Colleen Elmer,
M.S.W., M.B.A., LCSW

M. Colleen Elmer, M.S.W., M.B.A., LCSW, Executive Vice President & Senior Associate, brings twenty years of experience as an administrator, educator, and clinician. She has worked with a myriad of organizations including: state and local governments, pharmaceutical companies, managed care organizations, neurotechnology companies, and behavioral health and social services providers. Her projects have included strategic planning, clinical and operations reviews, marketing and business development, process reengineering, human resource management and succession planning, as well as a variety of large research projects.

Ms. Elmer served in senior management positions within the long-term care industry including Administrator and Director of Assisted Living Services at Messiah Village, Inc. in Pennsylvania. During her tenure as Administrator, the facility was deficiency-free on all inspections and received JCAHO accreditation. Ms. Elmer also created specialties in assisted living, including two levels of dementia care, respite, and hospice and redesigned all nursing care units into home-like neighborhoods. Ms. Elmer is certified as a Retirement Housing Professional at the Fellow level. She also served on a PANPHA subcommittee that helped define Assisted Living in Pennsylvania and recommended changes to the state on Assisted Living regulations.

Ms. Elmer served on faculty of Eastern University in both the Masters of Health Care Administration and MBA programs. She was involved in the re-design of the Health Care Administration program, including writing the curricula for managed care, long-term care/aging, issues in management, and health care informatics courses. She has also been a guest lecturer at Messiah College, Temple University, and Shippensburg University. Ms. Elmer has been a featured speaker for the Pennsylvania Adult Day Care Association, the Pennsylvania Association for Non-Profit Homes for the Aged, the American Association of Homes and Services for the Aged, the National Council for Community Behavioral Health Care and the National Association of Addiction Treatment Providers.

Her volunteer work includes serving on the board of directors of a local MR/DD group home, and the Cumberland County drug and alcohol commission. Ms. Elmer obtained her Bachelor's degree in Social Work from Messiah College, her Master's degree in Social Work from Temple University, and her Master's in Business Administration from Eastern University. She is also a Licensed Clinical Social Worker. ☒

Contributing Author

Niels T. Eskelsen, M.B.A., C.P.A.

Niels T. Eskelsen, M.B.A., C.P.A., Advisory Board Member, specializes in strategic business planning, management consulting, business and revenue development, business merger and acquisition, organizational reengineering, interim general and financial management. He has an extensive hands-on background in business management and consultation with over 30 years of experience in health care and industry organizations as an executive and business consultant. He is currently employed as the Director of Administration for Piedmont Area Behavioral Health in North Carolina. ☒

Contributing Author & Editor

J. Jay Mackie, Ph.D.

J. Jay Mackie, Ph.D., Associate Professor, Department of Accounting and Management Information Systems, Shippensburg University, earned his B.S. in accounting from Bentley College, an MBA from Northeastern University, and a Ph.D. in accounting from Texas A&M University.

His background includes over twenty five years of experience in both academic and business settings with areas of expertise in financial accounting, cost management, healthcare financial management, and business information systems. Dr. Mackie's current research interests involve accounting information systems, information technology, strategic cost management issues, and product costing in the health care industry. He is an advisory board member for the Institute for Behavioral Health Informatics and serves on the Shippensburg

University Health Care Administration degree completion program committee. He has published in Management Accounting, Journal of Accounting Education, Behavioral Health Management, *OPEN MINDS*, and The Pennsylvania CPA Journal. He has made numerous presentations at national and international conferences and is also the author of numerous monographs, book chapters, and newsletter articles related to the health care and social services field. ▩

Contributing Author

Joseph P. Naughton-Travers, Ed.M.

Joseph P. Naughton-Travers, Ed.M., Senior Associate, has over 20 years experience in the behavioral health and child welfare field. He has been a lead consultant with *OPEN MINDS* since 1998 and previously served as editor of its publications.

In his career, Mr. Naughton-Travers has had a broad range of experience in private and public sector delivery of behavioral health and social services. He started his career as a behavioral health clinician, working in both child welfare and community mental health clinic settings. Subsequently, Mr. Naughton-Travers held a senior business operations management position for a psychiatric hospital system and its community mental health clinics. Later, he was vice president of a firm specializing in management information systems and billing and receivables management for community-based mental health programs.

Mr. Naughton-Travers has provided consultation to provider and professional organizations, state and county government, technology companies, and venture capital firms. His primary areas of expertise include strategic planning and management, market research and analysis, operations improvement, OIG and HIPAA compliance, and information system technology. His specialty areas of focus within information technology include all components of IT system selection, (identifying functional specifications, RFP design, vendor selection and contracting), implementation, and IT Department structure and staffing. He has written numerous magazine articles on topics of interest to behavioral health and social service organizations, including "Winning the Human Resource Wars: Tried, True, & New Strategies For Behavioral Health and Social Service Organizations," "Five Pillars of Management Competency," "Data Driven

Decision Making: Moving to an Organizational Measurement Culture," and "HIPAA Administrative Simplification Round Two: Preparing For Compliance With Security Standards." He is also a nationally recognized speaker, having conducted hundreds of executive and professional executive training events around the nation. His primary areas of expertise include strategic planning and management, market research and analysis, operations improvement, OIG and HIPAA compliance, and information system technology. He received his Bachelor's degree from Miami University of Ohio and his Master's of Education in Counseling Psychology from Boston University. ▨

Contributing Author & Editor

Monica E. Oss, M.S.

Monica E. Oss, M.S., Chief Executive Officer and Senior Associate, is the founder of *OPEN MINDS*. Ms. Oss is a featured speaker on and author of numerous books and articles on industry trends and strategic marketing and management issues. She leads the *OPEN MINDS* consulting practice and serves as executive editor of its three information services. Ms. Oss has a broad range of executive experience in both the private and public sectors of the behavioral health and social service fields. Prior to *OPEN MINDS*, she was founder of a managed behavioral health program, vice president of a U.S. health risk management and underwriting division of an international insurance company, and head of account management for an occupational health services firm.

Ms. Oss has addressed dozens of national associations and affinity groups in the field including: the National Association of Addiction Treatment Providers; the American Psychological Association; the Child Welfare League of America; the National Community Behavioral Healthcare Council; and the National Alliance of the Mentally Ill. She has also served as the chairperson of the behavioral health track of the National Managed Health Care Congress and chaired the judging committee of the Eli Lilly Behavioral Healthcare Leadership Award.

Ms. Oss has led a range of industry research and management consultation initiatives, serving as principal investigator on research projects that included examination of managed behavioral health enrollment, employee assistance program models, rural mental health delivery models, and HMO behavioral health benefits plans. In addition, she has provided strategic consultation to provider and professional organizations, advocacy initiatives, state and county government agencies, pharmaceutical companies, technology companies, and venture capital firms.

Ms. Oss is a graduate of the University of Minnesota and has completed her doctoral course work in marketing and health care policy at George Washington University. She serves on the advisory boards of the Shippensburg University Health & Human Service Management Program, the Institute for Behavioral Health Informatics, and DrugRisk Solutions. She has previously served on numerous boards and advisory committees, including that of her local county's mental health/mental retardation oversight board and a regional Head Start program. ⅏

Contributing Author

John F. Talbot, Ph.D.

John F. Talbot, Ph.D., Executive Vice President and Senior Associate, has over 30 years experience in all aspects of health care, including upper management, consultation, education, direct clinical work, and serving as the president of a non-profit board. Dr. Talbot has provided consultation, training and operational assistance to behavioral health providers, nonprofit organizations, and managed care organizations across the country. Areas of focus for consultation and training include strategic planning, the development of successful strategic alliances, board development, organizational reengineering, operations management, management and leadership development, and change management.

Prior to his current position, Dr. Talbot served as the President of a network of agencies providing care to children and families. The innovative work of Colorado Care Management received national recognition, including participating in a Federal IV-E waiver study that demonstrated measurable superior clinical outcomes. In his role with Colorado Care Management, Dr. Talbot also led the development of a coalition of Colorado business executives to address the issues of providing care to abused and neglected children, and the establishment of a nationwide purchasing cooperative for non-profits. Dr.

Talbot's previous experience included serving as the Director of the Master of Health Systems Program, and Associate Dean of University College at the University of Denver. He also held senior management positions at Mount Airy Psychiatric Center, in Denver, Colorado.

Dr. Talbot has been a featured speaker at a number of national and state venues including the National Council Community Behavioral Health, Mental Health Corporations of America, the American Association of Residential Treatment Centers, the Medical Group Management Association, the Colorado Behavioral Health Council, the Mental Health Council of Arkansas, the New Jersey Association of Mental Health Agencies, and the Florida Behavioral Health Council.

Dr. Talbot is the former publisher and editor of Today's Healthcare Manager, a newsletter focusing on leadership and management skills for healthcare managers, and has written numerous articles, manuals, and book chapters. His volunteer work includes serving as the President of the Board of Human Services, Inc., in Colorado. ◙

About *OPEN MINDS*

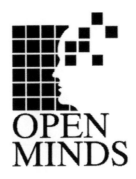

About *OPEN MINDS*

OPEN MINDS is a national behavioral health and social service industry market research and management consulting firm. Our mission is to provide executives in the field with the management knowledge and management tools necessary to create "best value" for consumers by facilitating the development of effective systems for financing and delivering service.

Founded in 1987 and based in Gettysburg, Pennsylvania, *OPEN MINDS* provides information, professional education, market research, and management consulting services to payers, regulators, professionals, service provider agencies, and advocacy organizations in the field. We provide the information that leads to better payer decisions and better provider delivery systems that, ultimately, lead to better behavioral health and social services for consumers.

OPEN MINDS offers customers three primary services in the behavioral health and social service field:

- Industry research and management consultation services
- Industry information products and services
- Professional development programs for executives, board members, managers, and professionals

Visit www.openminds.com for more information about *OPEN MINDS*. ◙

Mission

The mission of *OPEN MINDS* is to provide behavioral health, public health, and social service payers and provider organizations, and the vendor organizations that serve them with the market and management knowledge needed to improve their organizational efficiency and effectiveness.

Payers

Payers (whether corporations or managed care organizations or insurers or state governments…) are experiencing tremendous budget problems. Those customers are looking for ways to "hold the line" on spending (without reducing quality) in such areas as mental health services, chemical dependency treatment, drug testing, employee assistance, child protective services, services for the mentally-retarded and developmentally-disabled, long-term care services, and juvenile justice.

Payers' Issues: How to get "value" for the dollars they spend? How to control costs?

Our Role: Help to provide payers with the information needed to make these tough decisions.

Consumers

Consumers of behavioral health and human services are also facing challenging issues in this era of privatization, managed care, and health care reform. As the delivery systems change, consumers want information about how to get the services they need out of these new systems. These consumers are as diverse as the person who suffers from depression, the mother with an alcoholic son, the employee whose family problems are interfering with their work, the family with a profoundly retarded daughter, foster parents, and nursing home residents.

Consumers' Issues: How do I get the services I need in these new delivery systems? How can I tell if those services are "good"? What can I do to advocate for improvements in the system?

Our Role: Help consumers find answers to these questions.

Providers

Providers, the professionals and organizations that provide behavioral health and social services, include hospitals, physicians, psychologists, social workers, counselors, nurses, outpatient treatment programs, group practices, residential treatment facilities, group homes, case workers, probation officers, nursing homes, community mental health centers, managed care programs, and community-based programs. Never have providers of service faced such financial, operational, and ethical challenges as funding for services are restructured.

Providers' Issues: What business strategy is needed to adapt to this era of rapid change? What market information is needed to compete? What are the acceptable performance benchmarks for quality? For productivity? For pricing?

Our Role: To assist providers in obtaining the necessary information to answer these questions. ⊠

Industry Research & Management Consultation Services

Over the past two decades, *OPEN MINDS* team of researchers and consultants has provided research and management consulting support to over 200 organizations in the behavioral health and social service field. Our customer organizations include an array of behavioral health and social service professional service organizations: care management organizations, HMOs and insurance organizations, professional associations, and state/county/municipal government entities. The majority of our practice is based in the continental United States, with additional client organizations in Canada and Israel.

The *OPEN MINDS* research and consulting team brings its clients an experienced group of senior executives with a broad range of professional specialties. Our team is focused in developing and implementing practical solutions to today's most pressing management problems in the field. The team brings expertise in strategic planning, leadership development, governance, marketing and development, financial management, information technology, operations management, human resources, and new program development and implementation.

OPEN MINDS web site contains more information about the consulting practice and biographies of all consultants and advisory board members. Visit www.openminds.com/consult/researchconsulting.htm for details. ◨

Industry Information Products & Services

OPEN MINDS information products are its oldest and most widely known. The company began operations in April 1988 with the publication of the first issue of *OPEN MINDS, The Behavioral Health & Social Service Industry Analyst*, the company's flagship monthly newsletter. *OPEN MINDS* information products and services are developed by consultant experts from across the spectrum of the behavioral health and social service fields, covering all the key concepts outlined in this publication.

Subscriber services include a monthly management newsletter, weekly web-based news service, and a daily public-sector procurement notification e-mail service. The newest of our subscriptions services is the addition of *The OPEN MINDS Circle* – our award-winning, national on-line network of more than 12,000 executives, policy makers, and clinical professional responsible for the management and delivery of behavioral health and social services. It is the "go to" place and one-stop resource to find market intelligence and best practice management solutions for any range of behavioral health or human service programs – mental health, addictive disorders, child and family, child welfare, disability support, and long-term care. Basic membership in *The OPEN MINDS Circle* is free with options for a premium upgrade.

In addition to weekly news headlines of all the recent developments in the field, "hot topic" management articles, and updates on the latest contract awards, basic membership in *The OPEN MINDS Circle* contains an interactive "Ask the Expert" information exchange with on-line advice straight from the *OPEN MINDS* consulting team and executives from across the country. Also included is a Discussion Board – a place to share opinions, experience, or insight into pressing issues.

The Circle's full-text search function, powered by Google, queries over 20 years of resources found in *The OPEN MINDS Circle Library* – best practice management articles, profiles of the biggest and best companies, statistical report summaries, past news stories, white papers, government reports, and presentations from *OPEN MINDS* education events. All members use the

Google search to locate over 15,000 resources. Full access to all resources is allotted for premium members; basic members have restricted access to a smaller number of resources.

In addition to its subscriber services and products, *OPEN MINDS* produces a wide variety of other resources:
- Specialty datasets and survey research databases
- Industry mailing lists and databases
- Specialty and customer publications

To join *The OPEN MINDS Circle* or obtain additional details about *OPEN MINDS* publications and services, visit www.openminds.com/circle.htm. ◙

Management Development & Education Programs

One of the wisest investments an executive can make is in keeping management his or her skills updated, and there are few better ways to accomplish that than by attending *OPEN MINDS* executive events. Our events are designed for the busy executive to provide a fast track of essential business knowledge, up-to-the-minute industry information, and management skill development needed for health and human service executives to succeed in today's changing environment.

OPEN MINDS has over 15 years of experience conducting executive education events in all aspects of the health & human service field. Our event curriculum includes cutting-edge methods & processes, in-depth information on industry trends, and best practice models for executives in the key areas of the five pillars listed in this publication.

The newest addition to our event lineup is *OPEN MINDS Live & On-Line* webinar series. This series of on-line management seminars address cutting edge management topics in the health & human service field. Webinars are certified for the Shippensburg University of Pennsylvania Certificate in Health Care and Human Services Management and credentials for the American College of Addiction Treatment Administrators (ACATA). Each webinar session is a two-hour course on specific management topics. Each session includes a 90-minute presentation and a 30-minute interactive component for questions.

For a list of upcoming events, agendas, faculty, and sponsors, please visit *OPEN MINDS* web site at www.openminds.com/educ/calendar.htm. ⊠

2948413